EXAM PRIMER

Ready Revision

Series 2

LATHA VENKATESAN

VitMed
An Imprint of
Vitasta Publishing Pvt Ltd

Published by
VitMed
An Imprint of Vitasta Publishing Pvt Ltd
2/15, Ist Floor, Ansari Road,
Daryaganj, New Delhi-110 002
info@vitastapublishing.com

ISBN: 978-93-82711-84-1

Typesetting and Layout by Vitasta Publishing
Printed by Vit Press, New Delhi

This book is dedicated to all the nursing students,
who are the constant motivators for all the faculty

Contents

Preface

Butterflies in the stomach and worrying thoughts—'Will I be able to answer the questions?' 'Have I done enough revision?'—are indications of exam tensions that are probably familiar to all students. There are a number of things you can do to help manage exam anxiety and turn uncomfortable, panicky thoughts into more creative tension. This exam primer series is written to fill a vital need of the nursing students and nursing professionals to prepare themselves and perform well in qualifying examinations. The series includes 2 marks questions for all the subjects based on the INC syllabus for B.Sc nursing and PB B.Sc nursing courses. The two mark questions will also be helpful for the faculty involved in teaching nursing students in schools/colleges of nursing to prepare their students to score well in the exams. This series is written in a simple language and lucid style covering the subjects required by student nurses, keeping in view of the latest content and developments in pre clinical sciences and all specialties of nursing.

Apart from preparing the students for examination, this series also aims to help them in rapid and comprehensive revision of various subjects in nursing sciences. The questions and their answers have been thoroughly and repeatedly checked by the experts, but we shall refrain from claiming perfection. We shall deeply appreciate if such inadvertent omissions as well as suggestions for improvement of future editions are conveyed to us.

Acknowledgement

I am indebted to the nursing students who motivated me to compile this book by presenting their need for such a book to help them succeed in qualifying examinations. This edition of Exam Primer would not have been possible without the contributions of many nursing experts.

I thank all those whose comments and suggestions about the manuscript led to this collaborative effort by an outstanding group of contributors. Their expertise and knowledge of current nursing practice and management have added to the relevancy and accuracy of the material presented and they deserve special recognition for their continuing efforts.

DR. LATHA VENKATESAN

List of Contributors

Lizy Sonia, Vice Principal, Apollo College of Nursing, Chennai

Helen M, Associate Professor in Community Health Nursing, Apollo College of Nursing, Chennai

Jaslina Gnanarani, Associate professor in Medical Surgical Nursing, Apollo College of Nursing, Chennai

Sasikala, Associate Professor in Medical Surgical Nursing, Apollo College of Nursing, Chennai

Kanchana, Associate Professor in Medical Surgical Nursing, Apollo College of Nursing, Chennai

Abbreviations

AYUSH	Ay – Ayurveda, U – Unani, S – Siddha, H – Homeopathy
A.V AIDS	Audio Visual Aids
ASHA	Accredited Social Health Activist
AIDS	Acquired Immune Deficiency Syndrome
ACS	Acute Coronary Syndrome
ARI	Acute Respiratory Infection
ANM	Auxiliary Nurse Midwife
ACD	Acid Citrate Dextrose
ANP	Applied Nutri¬tion Programme
BCG	Bacilli Calmette-Guerin
BFHI	Baby Friendly Hospital Initiatives
BPH	Benign Prostatic Hyperplasia
BMI	Body Mass Index
BOAA	Beta Oxalyl Amino Alanine
BUN	Blood Urea Nitrogen
BHC	Benzene Hexachloride
CSW	Commercial Sex Worker
CPR	Couple Protection Rate.
CSSM	Center For The Study Of Society And Medicine
CAPD	Continuous Ambulatory Perito¬neal Dialysis
CHD	Coronary Heart Disease
CARE	Co-Operative American Relief Everywhere
CAM	Complementary And Alternative Medicine
CSF	Cerebrospinal Fluid
CRY	Child Relief And You
CMR	Crude Marriage Rate
CVA	Cardio Vascular Accident
CVD	Cardiovascular Diseases
COPD	Chronic Obstructive Lung Disease
DWCRA	Development Of Women And Children In Rural Area
DDS	Doctor Of Dental Surgery
DDT	Dichlorodiphenyltrichloroethane.
DPAP	Drought Prone Areas Program
DB	Decibels
DALY	Dis¬ability Adjusted Life Years
DOTS	Directly Observed Treatment Short Course

DES	Diethylstilbestrol
DEO	District Educational Officer
DUB	Dysfunctional Uterine Bleeding
DHA	Docosa Hexanoic Acid
DM	Diabetes Mellitus
ESI ACT	Employees' State Insurance Act
ELISA	Enzyme Linked Immunosorbant Assay
EDTA	Ethylene-Diamineteraacetic Acid
EPA	Environmental Protection Agency
FPAI	Family Planning Association Of India
FAO	Food And Agricultural Organization
FAT	Frans Activating Gene
FISH	Fluorescence In Situ Hybridization
GRR	Gross Reproductive Rate
GERD	Gastro Intestinal Esophageal Reflux Disease
GFR	Glomerular Filtration Rate
HAV	Hepatitis A Virus
HKNS	Hind Kusht Nivaran Sangh
HDLC & LDLC	High-Density Lipoprotein Cholesterol & Low -Density Lipoprotein Cholesterol
HTST METHOD	High Temperature And Short Time Method
HHNS	Hyperglycemic Hyperosmolar Nonketotic Syndrome
HCG	Human Chronic Gonadotropin
HBO	Hyperbaric Oxygen.
IMNCI	Integrated Management Of Neonatal And Childhood Illnesses
IG	Immunoglobulin
I.C.C.W	Indian Council For Child Welfare
IM INJECTION	Intramuscular Injection
IUD	Intrauterine Contraceptive Device
DSM DIAGNOSIS	Diagnostic And Statistical Manual Of Mental Disorders
IVP	Intravenous Pyelogram
JRC	Junior Red Cross.
JRYP	Jawahar Rozgar Yojana Programme
LH	Luteinizing Hormone
ICDS PROGRAMME	Integrated Child Development Services Programme
IV	Intravascular Injection
IRDP	Integrated Rural Development Programme
MAC	Mycobacterium Avium Complex
MCH SERVICES	Mean Corpuscular Hemoglobin Services
MTP	Medical Termina¬tion Of Pregnancy.
MMR	Maternal Mortality Rate
MDMP	Mid Day Meal Programme
MFAL	Marginal Farmers And Agricultural Laborers Project
NOA	Non-Obstructive Azoospermia
NMCP	National Malaria Control Programme
NMR	Neonatal Mortality Rate
NREP	National Rural Employment Programme

NRHM	National Rural Health Mission
NRR	Net Reproductive Rate
NSS	Nephron-Sparing Surgery
NSS	National service scheme
NCC	Non compaction Cardiomyopathy
NCC	National Cadet Corps
OPV	Oral Poliovirus Vaccine
PSA	Prostate Specific Antigen-A Glycoprotein
PCOD	Polycystic Ovarian Disorder
PRAI	Planning Research And Action Institute
PHC	Primary Hepatic Carcinoma
PEM	Protein Energy Malnutrition
PMR	Perinatal Mortality Rate
PPD	Purified Protein Derivative
PACU	Post Anesthesia Care Unit
PAT	Pre Admission Testing
PPFA	Planned Parenthood Federation Of America
PTH	Parathyroid Hormone
RA	Rheumatoid Arthritis
RTI	Reproductive Tract Infections
RCS	Reconstructive Surgery
RCA TYPE	Right Coronary Artery
RBC	Red Blood Cells
RLEP	Rural Landless Employment Guarantee Programme
SFDP	Small Farmers Development Project
STD	Sexually Transmitted Disease
SITRA	Supply Of Improved Tool Kits To Rural Artisans
SIMV	Synchronized Intermittent Mandatory Ventilation
SC	Subcutaneous
SLE	Systemic Lupus Erythematosis
SIADH	Syndrome Of Inappropriate Antidiuretic Hormone
TAI	Tuberculosis Association Of India
TRYSEM	Training Of Rural Youth For Self Development
TORCH	Toxoplasma Gondii, Other Viruses (HIV, Measles, And So On), Rubella (German Measles), Cytomegalovirus, And Herpes Simplex
TB	Tuberculosis
TLV	Time Threshold Limit Value
TPN	Trans Urethral Ultra Sound Guided Laser Induced Prostatectomy
TRYSEM	Training Rural Youth For Self Employment
TURP	Trans Urethral Resection Of Prostate
TUIP	Tran Urethral Incision Of Prostate
TWA	Time Weighted Average
TIPS	Transjugular Intrahepatic Portosys¬temic Shunt
UNICEF	United Nations International Emergency Fund
UHT	Ultra High Tempera¬ture
UV	Ultra Violet Radiation
VHAI	Voluntary Health Association Of India
VAD	Ventricular Assist Devices
WBC	White Blood Cells
WHO	World Health Organization.

COMMUNITY HEALTH NURSING

INTRODUCTION

Community has an influence on the health status of people. A community is a group of people living together in a particular geographical area or having the same culture or being associated with each other on the basis of education, occupation etc.

Community health nurses provide promotive, curative and rehabilitative service to the people. They provide services directly to individual, family and community.

The main factors affecting health care are:

- Human biology
- External environment
- Socio economic factors
- Availability of health services
- Social support system

Health promotion

Presently there is an increasing trend towards improving the quality of life rather than towards the traditional approach of disease control in the health field. Health promotion means making use of measures to improve the overall health status.

Health maintenance strategies

Following are the health maintenance strategies

- Nutrition
- Exercise
- Hygiene
- Stress reduction

- Health services
- Safe environment

Environment

Environment comprises all external condition that affects the life of an organism, the natural habitat aggregate that surrounds an organism.

Environmental pollution affects living as well as non- living components. It affects the health of human beings and animals and also damages property and plants.

Social structure

Every society has a social structure. Social structure is the pattern of inter relations between individuals. Each individual in the society acquires beliefs, customs and traditions in his everyday social interactions.

Hygiene is maintained to preserve health. It has two aspects— environmental hygiene and personal hygiene. A number of factors are associated with hygienic practices. Unhygienic practices lead to several health problems.

Epidemiology

Epidemiology is concerned with the improvement of health. Epidemiology has provided new opportunities for prevention, control, treatment and improvement of health services.

Demography

Demography is the study of human population in terms of size, structure and distribution. Demography provides a tool to approach a large range of population issues by combining a more technical quantitative approach. Demographic data is presented in terms of rate and ratio such as birth rate, death rate, etc.

Arthropods borne diseases are major health problems. These are transmitted by direct contact, mechanically and biologically. There is a need to control arthropod borne diseases by adopting appropriate strategies such as using antilarval measures, antiadult control measures and protection against mosquito bites.

Food hygiene means all measures adopted during production, processing, storing and distribution of food, to make food safe and wholesome. Food should be handled and stored in a proper way. Food additives are used to preserve the food for a prolonged time period. Food poisoning can occur due to unhygienic food consumption. Adulterated food, if consumed produces many effects on health.

References

1. Kumari N. (2009). **A Textbook of Community Health Nursing.** Ist ed. Vikas & Co.
2. Park K (2013). **Textbook of Preventive and Social medicine.** 21th ed. M/S Banarsidas Bhanot.
3. Kamalam S (2005). **Essentials in Community Health Nursing Practice.** 1st ed. Jaypee.

Test Series I

1. **Define Eugenics.**
   Eugenics is the science which aims to improve the genetic endowment of the human population.
2. **Elaborate AYUSH.**
   Ay – Ayurveda, U – Unani, S – Siddha, H – Homeopathy.
3. **Define BMI.**
   BMI is Body Mass Index which is simple index of weight for height and it is commonly used to classify underweight, overweight & obesity in adults.
   BMI = Weight in Kg/Height in cm2
4. **Define epidemiology.**
   It is defined as "The study of distribution and determinants of health related status and events in specified populations and the application of this study to the control of health problems".
5. **Define quarantine.**
   It has been defined as, "the limitation of freedom of movement of such well persons or domestic animals exposed to communicable disease for a period of time not longer than the usual incubation period of the disease, in such manner as to prevent effective contact with those not so exposed.
6. **Define immunity.**
   Immunity is the resistance possessed by the body to infectious diseases, foreign tissue, foreign nontoxic substances and others.
7. **Define environment.**
   "The term environment implies all the external factors living and nonliving, material and nonmaterial which surrounds man.
8. **Define food fortification.**
   Fortification of food is a public health measure aimed at reinforcing the usual dietary intake of nutrients with additional supplies to prevent/control some nutritional disorder and to improve the quality of the diet of a group or a community or a population. E.g. Iodised salt to prevent goiter.
9. **Define health promotion.**
   Health promotion is the process of enabling people to increase control over and to improve their health. It moves beyond a focus on individual behaviour towards a wide range of social and environmental interventions.
10. **Define population medicine.**
   Population medicine is referred to as hygiene, public health, preventive medicine and social medicine or community medicine. All these share common ground in their concern for promotion of health and

prevention of diseases.

11. Define rehabilitation.

It is defined as "the combined and coordinated use of medical, social, educational and vocational measures for training and retraining the individual to the highest possible level of functional ability.

12. Define weaning.

Weaning is a process of introducing supplement foods to a suckling infant. The process begins when weaning foods are given along with breast feeding and ends when the baby is completely taken off the breast.

13. Mention the objectives of sub centre.

- To provide mother & child health care.
- To promote family planning services.
- To promote immunization coverage.

14. Name the communicable diseases caused by bacteria.

- **Acute diarrhoeal diseases** – E coli, Shigella.
- **Tuberculosis** – Mycobacterium tuberculosis.
- **Diphtheria** –Diptheriae.
- **Whooping Cough** – B. Pertusis.
- **Cholera** – V. cholerae.
- **Typhoid** – S. typhi.

15. List the steps involved in conducting community programme.

- Analyse the health situation.
- Establish goals and objectives.
- Assessment of resources.
- Fixing priorities.
- Write up formulated plan.
- Programming and implementation.
- Monitoring and evaluation.

16. List the functions of gram panchayat.

- It is the agency for planning and development at village level.
- Civic administration.
- Promote sanitation and public health.
- Economic development of village.

17. Mention the three main functions of central council of India.

- Health policy making.
- Public health legislation.
- To promote and maintain co-operation between Central and State Health Administration.

18. List the six interconnected links of infection transmission.

- Pathogenic agent
- Reservoir
- Portal exit
- Mode of transmission
- Portal of entry
- Host susceptibility

19. List few family focused interventions.

- Health screening
- Lifestyle modification
- Health education
- Counselling
- Primary health care
- Immunization
- Social support etc

20. List the ethical principles in health care.

- Autonomy
- Respect for persons
- Beneficence
- Non-maleficence
- Justice
- Veracity
- Fidelity
- Written consent

21. Mention few occupational diseases.

- Pneumoconiosis
- Lead poisoning
- Occupational cancer
- Occupational dermatitis
- Carbon disulphide poisoning

- Carbon monoxide poisoning
- Insecticide poisoning
- Hearing impairment
- Diseases of agricultural workers

22. Mention the effect of population growth.

- Socio-economic effects.
- Biological effects.
- Effects on health.

23. List important causes of infant mortality in India.

- Low birth weight.
- Diarrhoeal diseases.
- Acute respiratory tract infection.
- Malnutrition.
- Congenital abnormalities.
- Accidents.
- Other communicable diseases.

24. List the health problems due to industrialization.

- Environmental sanitation problem.
- Communicable disease problem.
- Food and sanitation problem.
- Problems of mental health or mental illness.
- Accident.
- Social problem.

25. List down the uses of epidemiology.

- To study historically about the rise and fall of disease in the population.
- Plan for Community diagnosis.
- Planning and evaluation.
- Evaluation of individual risks and chances.
- Syndrome identification.
- Completing the natural history of disease.
- Searching for causes and risk factors.

26. List down the aims of epidemiology.

- To describe the distribution and magnitude of health and disease problems in population.
- To identify etiological factors.
- To provide the data essential for the planning, implementation and evaluation of services for the prevention, control and treatment of diseases.

27. Elaborate the ABCDEF of nutritional assessment.

A - Anthropometric
B - Biochemical examination
C - Clinical examination
D - Dietary assessment
E - Evaluation of ecology factor
F - Functional assessment

28. What are the maternity benefits under ESI Act.

- For confinement – 12 weeks leave.
- For miscarriage – 6 weeks leave.
- Sickness arising out of pregnancy – 4 weeks leave.
- Rate of benefit in full rate.

29. Mention the radical treatment of malaria.

P. Vivax – Tab. Primaquine – 0.25mg/kg body weight and 15 mg adult dose daily for 5 days.

P. Falciparum – Tab. Chloroquine 10mg/kg body weight plus tab. Primaquine 0.75 mg/kg body weight single dose.

30. What is herd immunity?

It is the level of resistance of a community or a group of people to a particular disease. It implies group protection beyond that afforded by the protection of immunized individuals.

31. Name the health workers at village level.

- Multipurpose health workers.
- Village health guides.
- Local dais.
- Anganwadi workers.
- Trained birth attendants.

- Skilled birth attendants.
- ASHA (Accredited Social Health Activist).
- Health assistants.

32. Mention components of RCH package.

- Family Planning.
- CSSM.
- Client approach to health care.
- Prevention/Management of RTI/STD/AIDS.

33. List aspects of school health services.

- Health appraisal of school children.
- Remedial measures and follow up.
- Prevention of communicable diseases.
- Healthful school environment.
- Nutritional services.
- First aid and emergency care.
- Mental health.
- Dental health.
- Eye health and health education.
- Education for handicapped children.
- Proper maintenance of school health records.

34. List down the scope of community health nurses in India.

- School Health Nurse.
- Geriatric Nurse.
- Home Health Care Nurse/Home Care.
- Industrial Nurse.
- Railway Nurses.
- Palliative Care Nurse.

35. List down the social security measures for industrial workers in India.

- Workmen's Compensation Act, 1923.
- Central Maternity Benefits Act, 1961.
- Employees State Insurance Act, 1948.
- The Family Pension Scheme, 1971.

36. Mention the two distinct types of analytical study.

- Case control study.
- Cohort study.

37. Who is the father of vital statistics?

John Gruant (1660-1674).

38. Who is the father of medical statistics?

William Farr (1807-1883)

39. List down the mass media methods in health education.

- Television.
- Radio, internet & newspaper.
- Printed materials (magazine, pamphlets).
- Direct mailing, posters, folk media.
- Museums & exhibitions.

40. Mention the scope of health education.

- Human biology.
- Family health.
- Disease prevention and control.
- Hygiene & nutrition.
- Mental health.
- Prevention of accidents, etc.

41. List down the disadvantages of bottle feeding.

- No bonding.
- No lactation amenorrhoea.
- Poor jaw development.
- Inconvenience for the mother.
- Risk of anemia.
- Risk of malnutrition.
- Risk for bottle addiction syndrome.
- Risk of getting infection.

42. List down the norms of weaning.

- Appreciating quality.
- Consistency should be gradual change.
- Safety – hygiene preparations.
- Suitability (Taste of the food).
- Frequency should be appropriate.

43. List down the objectives of BFHI.

Baby friendly hospital initiatives

- To enable mothers to make an informed choice about how to feed their

babies.
- To support early initiation of breast feeding.
- To promote exclusive breast feeding for the first 4-6 months.
- To discourage commercial infant milk substitutes.
- To avoid free milk substitutes to the hospitals.
- To include other infant care issues at a later date.

44. List behavioural problems in children.

Antisocial behaviour – Stealing, cruelty, sexual offense, destructiveness.
Education difficulties – Slow learner, school phobia, repeated failure.
Habit disorders – Bed wetting, nail biting, thumb sucking, masturbation.
Personality disorder – Jealous, hysteric.
Psychosomatic disorder – Delusion, depression, hallucinations.

45. List the advantages of breast feeding.

- Natural and convenient.
- It contains the requisite nutrition for the baby.
- It easily digestible and assimilable.
- It is economical and readily available.
- It prevents infections /increases immunity.
- It promotes bonding between mother and baby.
- Promotes optimal growth and development (physical and intellectual).
- Prevents malnutrition.
- Helps in early involution of the uterus.
- Breast feeding helps to delay subsequent child birth acting as a birth control measure.

46. List down the common problems of the mother during breast feeding.

- Flat or retracted nipple.
- Sore nipple.
- Breast engorged.
- Mastitis.
- Breast abscess.

47. List down the successive steps of rehabilitation.

- Assessment of the patient's physical, mental, socio-economic and vocational status.
- Diagnosis of the therapeutic, physio therapeutic, vocational, educational training, and supportive needs of the client.
- Deciding the minimum acceptable improvement in the patient's health capacity for independence, and productivity level.
- Formulating a plan of action to meet the decided minimum standards.
- Implementing the action plan.
- Evaluate the result of intervention.
- Modification of the plan of action, if necessary.

48. Expand the terms TRYSEM, SITRA, DWCRA, IRDP.

- TRYSEM – Training of Rural Youth for Self Development.
- SITRA – Supply of Improved Tool Kits to Rural Artisans.
- DWCRA – Development of Women and Children in Rural Area.
- IRDP – Integrated Rural Development Programme.

49. Define health

Health is a complete state of physical, mental, social wellbeing not merely the absence of disease or infirmity-WHO.

50. What is the other name of Heath Planning and Development Committee?

Bhore Committee – 1946.

Test Series II

1. **What are schemes for community development in India.**
   - 100 days working scheme.
   - Various educational schemes.
   - Health insurance scheme by Kalaignar Kapeetu Thittam.
   - Community development scheme e.g., Arignar Anna Scheme.
   - Improvement of housing standards etc.
   - Female child marriage scheme.
2. **Name the voluntary health agencies which work for children's right at national Level.**
   - Indian Council for Child Welfare.
   - Central Social Welfare Board.
   - Junior Red cross.
3. **Name some of the voluntary health agencies which work for children right at State Level.**
   - Udavi.
   - Annai Gandhi.
   - Udavum Karangal, etc.
4. **What is DOTS?**
   It is directly observed treatment short course chemotherapy. It is a strategy to ensure treatment of tuberculosis by providing most effective medicine and confirming that it is taken.
5. **When was NMCP launched, when was it renamed as national antimalarial Programme?**
   It was launched in the year 1953, and it was renamed as national anti malarial programme in the year 1999.
6. **What type of surgery is promoted to prevent disability in leprosy?**
   RCS – Reconstructive Surgery to improve the functional status of individuals who is affected by leprosy.
7. **What mono therapy is used in leprosy?**
   DDS (Dapsone) monotherapy is used in leprosy.
8. **Mention the single dose mass drug therapy for filarial.**
   Diethyl carbamazepine with albendazole.
9. **Define empowerment.**
   Empowerment is about people both men and women taking control over their bodies setting their own agenda, gaining skills, increasing self-confidence and solving their problems and developing self-reliance. It is both a process and an outcome.
10. **List down the principles of PHC.**
    - Equitable distribution.
    - Intersectoral co-ordination.
    - Community participation.

- Appropriate technology.
- Manpower development.

11. Mention the five causes of MTP.

- Medical
- Eugenic
- Humanitarian
- Socio-economic
- Failure of contraceptive devices

12. List down the qualities of ASHA.

- A woman (Married/widow/divorced).
- Age 25 to 45 years.
- Resident of same village.
- Completed 8th standard of formal education.
- Should have good communication and leadership skills.

13. Define community.

"A community is a social group determined by geographical boundaries and or common values and interests. Its members know and interact with each other.

14. Define culture.

It is defined as "Learned behaviour which has been socially acquired and it is transmitted from one generation to another generation through learning processes-formal and informal. It plays an imparted fact in human societies.

15. Define sanitation.

Sanitation is the "scheme of safeguarding health." It is a way of life, it is the quality of living that is expressed in the clean home, the clean farm, clean business, the clean neighbourhood and the clean community.

16. Define environmental sanitation.

It is defined as "the control of all those factors in man's physical environment which exercise or may exercise a deleterious effect on his physical development, health and survival.

17. What is the purpose of environmental sanitation?

To create and maintain ecological conditions that will promote health and thus prevent disease.

18. List down the functions of air.

- It supplies the life by giving oxygen.
- Making human body cool and comfortable.
- Helpful in hearing and smell functions through air transmitted stimuli.
- Adequate air circulation prevent disease transmission.

19. List down the determinants of health.

Individual determinants: Aging of the population, sociocultural, sciences and technology.

Family determinants: Gender, information and communication equity and social justice.

Societal determinants: Environmental, socio-economic, health system.

Community determinants: Human rights, biological, behavioural.

20. Define positive eugenics.

It seeks to improve the genetic composition of the population by encouraging the carrier of desirable genotypes of assume the burden of parenthood. E.g. determination of gene transmission.

21. List down requirements of good lighting.

- Sufficiency
- Distribution
- Absence of glare
- Absence of sharp shadows
- Steadiness
- Colour of light
- Surroundings

22. What is sentinel surveillance?

No routine notification system can identify all cases of infection or disease. A method for identifying the missing cases and thereby supplementing the notified cases is required. This is known as sentinel surveillance.

23. Define natural history of disease.

Disease results from a complex interaction between man, an agent (or cause) and the environment. This is called natural history of disease. This is a key concept of epidemiology.

24. Name types of cohort studies.

- Prospective cohort studies.
- Retrospective cohort studies.
- Combination of both.

25. Define cold chain.

The cold chain is a system of storage and transport of vaccines at low temperature from the manufacture place to actual vaccination site.

26. Mention the two types of immunity.

Natural immunity

Acquired immunity.

27. List down the types of communication.

- One way communication.
- Two way communication.
- Verbal communication.
- Non verbal communication.
- Formal & informal communication.
- Visual communication, telecommunication and internet.

28. What are the hazards of radiation.

- Burns
- Dermatitis
- Blood dyscariasis
- Chronic exposure leads to malignancies
- Genetic defects
- Lung cancer

29. Enlist types of occupational hazards?

- Physical hazards (Heat, cold, light noise etc.).
- Chemical hazards (Metals, dusts, gases etc).
- Biological hazards (Brucellosis, leptospirosis, anthrax, etc).
- Mechanical hazards (Injury, fracture).
- Psychological hazards (Frustration, insecurity, lack of job satisfaction, emotional tension, etc).

30. What are components of under five clinic?

- Care in illness.
- Preventive care.
- Growth monitoring.
- Family planning.
- Health education.

31. Name components of MCH services.

- Maternal health
- Family planning
- Child health
- School health
- Care of handicapped children.
- Care of the children in special settings such as day care centres.

32. List down the indicators of MCH care.

Maternal mortality rate

Mortality in infancy and childhood

- Perinatal mortality rate.
- Neonatal mortality rate.
- Post neonatal mortality rate.
- Infant mortality rate.
- 1-4 years mortality rate.
- Under five mortality rate.
- Child survival rate.

33. Define health education.

"The process by which individuals and groups of people learn to behave in a manner conducive to the promotion, maintenance or restoration of health"

– John M. Last.

Health education is a process that informs,

motivates and helps people to adopt and maintain healthy practices and lifestyles, advocates environmental changes as needed to facilitate this goal and conducts professional training and research to the same end.

– National Conference on Preventive Medicine in USA.

It is the process aimed at encouraging people who want to be healthy, to know how to stay healthy, to do what they can individually and collectively to maintain health and to seek help when needed

– Alma Ata (1978)

34. Mention the modes of intervention.

- Health promotion.
- Specific protection.
- Easy diagnosis early & treatment.
- Disability limitation.
- Rehabilitation.

35. List down the determinants of fertility.

- Age at marriage.
- Duration of marriage.
- Spacing of children.
- Child survival.
- Educational status.
- Economic stability.
- Cultural belief and practices.

36. Write down the principles of fertility regulation.

- Avoid untimely pregnancies.
- Avoid too close pregnancies.
- Avoid too many pregnancies.
- Avoid unwanted pregnancies.
- Avoid risky pregnancies.

37. Mention the benefits of fertility regulation.

- Benefits to mother.
- Benefits to child.
- Benefits to family.
- Benefits to community and country.

38. List down the type of employment examination of any industrial workers.

Comprehensive health checkup includes age, height, weight, BP, heart rate, respiratory rate, hearing acuity, visual acuity, physical efficacy, vital capacity, productive capacity.

Periodical examination – Thorough physical examination, hematological, bacteriological, serological, parasitological and radiological investigations.

39. Define ergonomics.

It is a study of man at work, to identify two stress factors operating in working environment while imparting the physical, mental, psychological wellbeing of workers and interfering work performance. It is multidisciplinary such as psychology, anthropology, physiology, epidemiology, engineering bio mechanics etc.

40. Mention the problems of old age.

- **Problems due to aging:** physiological changes of age, e.g. changes in cells, tissues and organs, etc., e.g. visual impairment, skin changes etc.
- **Problems due to chronic illness,** e.g.: cancer, hypertension, diabetes, etc.
- **Psychological problems** like dementia, delirium etc. empty nest syndrome.
- **Social problem** like poverty, lifestyle changes etc.

41. Elaborate the five 'F' of disease transmission.

F – Food
F – Fomite
F – Finger
F – Flies
F – Faeces

42. Define eligible couple.

An eligible couple refers to a married couple

wherein the wife is in the reproductive age of 14-45yers.

43. Define disaster.

Disaster can be defined as "any occurrence that causes damage, ecological disruption, loss of human life".

44. When did baby friendly hospitals come into being?

These were established under the baby friendly hospital initiative, WHO and UNICEF launched at BFHI in 1991 at the International Pediatric Association Conference held at Ankara.

45. List down the signs and symptoms of breast engorgement.

- Fever
- Pain
- Tense and tender breast
- Knobby to feel

46. Name few institutions working for challenged children.

- All India Institute of Physical Medicine and Rehabilitation, Mumbai.
- All India Institute of Speech and Hearing, Mysore.
- Ali Yavar Jung National Institute for the Hearing Handicapped, Mumbai.
- Institute of Physical Medicine and Rehabilitation Centre, Vellore.
- National Institute for the Visually Handicapped, Dehradun.
- Occupational Therapy College, New Delhi.
- Physical Therapy School, Mumbai.
- Many other non-government voluntary organizations.

47. What is the concept of Ayurveda?

Tridosha concept: Vata (gas), pitta (gall), Kapha (mucus).

In equilibrium of three humors cause diseases in our body.

48. List down the main combination of Sidha medicine.

Mainly it is having mercury, silver, arsenic, lead and sulphur.

49. List down the diseases which may come under iceberg phenomena.

- Hypertension
- Diabetes Mellitus
- Malnutrition
- Mental Illness

50. List down the various approaches of health care.

- Hospital approach.
- Public health approach.
- Regulatory approach.
- Educational approach.
- Primary health care approach.
- Risk approach.
- Integrated approach.

Test Series III

1. **List down the components of evaluation of community programme.**
    - Relevancy
    - Cost efficacy
    - Progress
    - Effectiveness
    - Outcome
2. **List down the components of minimum needs programme.**
    - Rural health
    - Rural water supply
    - Rural electrification
    - Rural education
    - Adult education
    - Nutrition
    - Improvement of urban slums
    - Houses for landless labourers
3. **Enlist nutritional programmes in India.**
    - Vitamin A prophylaxis programme.
    - Nutritional anaemia prophylaxis programme.
    - Iodine deficiency disease control programme.
    - Special nutrition programme.
    - Balwadi nutrition programme.
    - ICDS programme.
    - Mid-day meal scheme programme.
    - Applied nutrition programme.
4. **List down stages of malaria.**
    - Cold stage – Headache, nausea, T=39-40°C.
    - Hot stage – Lasts for 2-6 hours. Skin is hot & dry.
    - Sweating stage – Skin is cold and moist. This stage lasts for 2-4 hours.
5. **Mention the three main clinical forms of plague.**
    - Bubonic plague.
    - Pneumonic plague.
    - Septicaemic plague.
6. **Define YAWS.**

    It is a chronic contagious non venereal disease caused by T.pertenue usually beginning in early childhood.
7. **Mention two kinds of confirmatory test for HIV**
    - ELISA
    - Western BLOT
8. **List three stages of cholera.**

    Stage of evacuation:
    - Profuse, painless, watery diarrhoea followed by vomiting 40 times a day.
    - Stage of collapse:
    - Sunken eyes, hollow cheeks, washerman's hands and feet, absent/unrecordable BP, loss of skin elasticity, shallow

and quick respirations, decreased urine output and death may occur.

Stage of recovery:

- If death does not occur, the patients begin to show clinical improvement.

9. Write down the types of Ventilation.

Natural Ventilation:

- The wind
- Diffusion
- Inequality of temperature

Artificial Ventilation:

- Exhaust ventilation
- Plenum ventilation
- Balanced ventilation
- Air conditioning

10. What are the methods of disinfection of air.

- **Mechanical ventilation** – Reduce the bacterial density.
- **Ultra violet radiation** – Effective in operation theatre.
- **Chemical mists** – Triethylene glycol vapours effective bactericides.
- **Dust control** – Application of oil to the floor.

11. List down the qualities of sanitary well.

- **Location** – Higher elevated position.
- **Lining** – By bricks/stones should be 2-3 feet, above ground level.
- **Parapet** – Parapet wall height 28 inches.
- **Platform** – Cement, concrete platform round the well at least in all the direction.
- **Drain** – Pucca drain to carry spilled water.
- **Covering** – Cement concrete cover.
- Hand pump – For lifting the water.
- **Consumer responsibility** – For cleanliness.
- **Quality** – Acceptable standard.

12. List down some water borne diseases.

- **Viral** – Viral hepatitis A, hepatitis E, poliomyelitis, rotavirus, diarrhoea.
- **Bacterial** – Typhoid and paratyphoid fever, bacillary dysentery, Esch. coli. diarrohea, cholera.
- **Protozoal** – Amoebiasis, giardiasis.
- Helminthic – Round worm, thread-worm, hydrated disease.
- **Leptospural** – Weil's disease.
- **Snail** – Schistosomiasis.
- **Cyclops** – Guinea worm, fish tape worm.

13. Define intervention in community.

Intervention can be defined as any attempt to intervene or interrupt the usual sequence in the development of disease in man. This may be the treatment, education, help or social support.

14. Mention five major classes of human immunoglobulin.

- Immunoglobulin G (IgG)
- Immunoglobulin M (IgM)
- Immunoglobulin A (IgA)
- Immunoglobulin D (IgD)
- Immunoglobulin E (IgE)

15. List down the hazards of immunization.

- Reaction inherent to inoculation – Pain swelling, redness, tenderness, abscess etc.
- Reaction due to faulty techniques – Streptococcal, staphylococcal infections.
- Reaction due to hypersensitivity reaction – Bronchospasm, dyspnea, pallor, hypotension, collapse etc.
- Neurological involvement – Encephalitis, Guillain-Barre Syndrome.
- Provocative reactions.

- Other damage to fetus.

16. List down the types of screening.

- Mass screening.
- High risk or selective screening.
- Multi phase screening.

17. Define gene therapy.

Gene therapy is the introduction of a gene sequence into a cell with the aim of modifying the cells behaviour in a clinically relevant fashion.

18. List down the health impact of improper waste management.

- Nuisance from bad odours.
- Water and soil pollution.
- Breeding place of flies and mosquitoes, etc.
- It attracts rodents and vermin.
- Spread of communicable diseases.

19. Define secondary attack rate in community.

It is defined as "the number of exposed person developing the disease within the range of the incubation period, following exposure to the primary care".

20. Define health.

According to WHO (1948) "Health is a state of complete physical, mental & social well-being and not merely the absence of disease or infirmity."

21. Define Community Health Nursing.

Community Health Nursing is a synthesis of nursing and public health practice applied to promoting the health of people. The practice is general and comprehensive.

The unique function of the nurse is to assist the individual, sick or well in the performance of those. Considers the biological, psychological, sociological, and spiritual components.

22. Define primary health care.

"Essential health care based on practical, scientifically sound and socially acceptable methods and technologically made universally accessible to individuals and families in the community through their full participation and at a cost that the community and the country can afford to maintain at every stage of their development in the spirit of self-determination".

23. Write about spectrum of health.

Positive health
Better health
Freedom from sickness

Unrecognized sickness
Mild sickness
Severe sickness
Death

24. Define primary health care.

"Essential health care based on practical, scientifically sound and socially acceptable methods and technologically made universally accessible to individuals and families in the community through their full participation and at a cost that the community and the country can afford to maintain at every stage of their development in the spirit of self-determination".

24. Define hygiene.

The word "Hygiene" is derived from Hygeia, the goddess of health in Greek mythology and it is defined as "the science of health and embraces all factors which contribute to healthful living".

25. Write down the various approaches of fertility regulation.

- Educational approach.
- Motivational approach.
- Integrated approach.

- Service approach.
- Legal approach.

26. Write down the different method of fertility regulation.

- Contraception
- Termination
- Sterilization

27. List down the side effects of oral contraceptive pills.

- **Minor effects like** – Nausea, vomiting, headache, breast tenderness, depression etc.
- **Menstrual changes** – Oligomenorrhoea/amenorrhoea.
- **Breast changes** – Heaviness, tenderness
- **Utero vaginal changes** – Congestion of ervix dysplasia etc.
- **Cardio vascular changes** – CHD, HT, CVD.
- **Hepatobiliary changes** – Cholestatic jaundice, cholecystitis.
- **Metabolic changes** –Increase the HDLC & LDLC.
- **Nutritional changes** – Suffering from borderline malnutrition.
- **Psychological changes** – Depression, loss of libido.
- Skin changes of chloasma on face and forehead.

28. List down the complications of pregnancy termination/abortion.

- Cervical injury.
- Uterine haemorrhage.
- Uterine perforation.
- Infection.
- Failure.

29. Explain socio-cultural impact upon health.

- Colostrum feeding is harmful in some culture where it may cause Protein Energy Malnutrition (PEM) in future. Consumption of fish and milk is believed to produce leucoderma.
- Pregnant women are advised for small meals to avoid a bigger sized baby.
- Drinking of buffalo milk by children is thought to blunt their intellect.
- Prolonged boiling of vegetables in open vessels and discarding of excess rice water, peeling of roots and tubers contribute a loss of various nutrients.

30. List common bacterial food poisoning.

- Salmonella food poisoning.
- Staphylococcal food poisoning.
- Botulism (by el. Botulinum).
- Clostridium perfringens food poisoning.

31. Write down the four aspects of behaviour development of children.

- Motor development.
- Personal and social development.
- Adaptive development.
- Language development.

32. List down the uses of growth chart.

- For growth monitoring.
- Diagnostic tool.
- For planning and policy making.
- Educational tool for mothers.
- Tools for action e.g., referrals.
- For evaluation purpose.

33. Name a few child related health problems in India.

- Low birth weight
- Malnutrition
- Infections and parasitosis /worm infestation
- Dental problems
- Skin problems
- Accidents and poisoning
- Behavioural problems

34. List down few occupational cancers.

- Skin cancer
- Lung cancer
- Cancer bladder
- Leukemia

35. List down the control measures of industrial cancers.

- Elimination or control of industrial carcinogens.
- Periodic medical examinations.
- Inspection of factories.
- Notification.
- Licensing of establishments.
- Personal hygiene measures.
- Education of workers.
- Research.

36. List occupational hazards of agricultural workers.

- **Zoonotic diseases** e.g.: Brucellosis, anthrax, leptospirosis, tetanus, tuberculosis (bovine).
- **Accidents** – By machinery, insect and snake bite, etc.
- **Toxic hazards** – By chemicals like fertilizers, insecticides and pesticides.
- **Physical hazards** – Heat stroke, sun burns etc.
- **Respiratory diseases** – Such as sinusitis, bagassosis, farmer's lung and occupational asthma..

37. List down the causes of accidents in industry.

- Poor physical capabilities of the worker
- Physiological factors like increased hormonal level.
- Psychological factors – Emotional stress, carelessness etc.
- Environmental factors such as poor illumination, humidity, noise and unsafe machines.

38. What is MMR?

It is the number of deaths from puerperal causes per 1000 live births in one year is termed Maternal Mortality Rate.

$$\text{MMR} = \frac{\text{No. of deaths from puerperal causes}}{\text{Total live births in the year}} \times 1000$$

The death occurring during pregnancy or within 42 days of the delivery.

39. Define nenotal mortality deat.

No. of neonatal deaths (death within 28 days of birth) per 1000 live births in one year.

$$\text{NMR} = \frac{\text{No. of deaths under 28 days of age}}{\text{Total live births in the year}} \times 1000$$

40. What is perinatal mortality?

It comprises late foetal deaths (still births) and early neonatal deaths e.g.:It includes deaths between 28th week of pregnancy and the end of 1st week after birth.

$$\text{PMR} = \left[\frac{\text{Late foetal deaths (28 weeksor more + death under 1 week}}{\text{Total live birth + still birth}}\right] \times 1000$$

weighing over1000 gms at birth

41. What are the 10 steps of successful breastfeeding recommended by BFHI.

- Draft a written breastfeeding policy and communicate it to all staff routinely.
- Train all staff in skills necessary to implement this policy.
- Inform all pregnant women about the management and benefits of breast feeding.
- Help mothers initiate breastfeeding within 30 minutes of birth.
- Show mothers how to breast feed, and how to maintain lactation even if they should be separated from their infant's part of the time.
- Do not give new born infants food and

drink other than breast milk unless medically indicated.
- Keep mothers and their baby together 24 hours of the day.
- Encourage mothers to breast feed the baby on demand.
- Do not give teats or pacifiers to the infant.
- Foster the establishment of breast feeding support groups. Refer mothers on discharge to one of these groups.

42. Mention few feeding reflexes.
- Rooting reflex
- Sucking reflex
- Swallowing reflex
- Gag reflex

43. Define vital statistics.

It is defined as the facts, systematically collected and compiled in numerical form, related to or derived from records of vital events. The vital events are legally registered. "Vital statistics is the collection, compilation, presentation analysis and distribution of statistics pertaining to vital events are recorded e.g., live birth, death, marriage.

44. Define status.

Status is a position which the individual occupies in the group by virtue of his age, sex, family, class, occupation, marriage and achievement.

45. List down few international agencies involved in child welfare.

UNICEF – United Nations International Emergency Fund.

WHO – World Health Organization.

CARE – Co-operative American Relief Everywhere.

FAO – Food and Agricultural Organization.

46. What are principles of complementary alternative medicine.
- The body has ability to heal itself.
- Health and healing are related to harmony to mind, body and spirit.
- Individuals are responsible for their own healing.

47. Name some of the body mind intervention in naturopathy.

Prayer, meditation, imagery, hypnosis, music/art therapy, journaling, animal assisted therapy etc.

48. Define moon survey.

The definitive diagnosis of lymphatic filariasis living parasites in the human body comes up to the capillary blood during the night time. So the blood is collected from deep finger prick between 10.00 PM and 12 mid night is called moon survey.

49. Mention the complication of filariasis.
- Painful swollen limbs with lymphoedema or elephantiasis.
- Hydrocele is common in males.

50. What is the symbol of under five clinic.

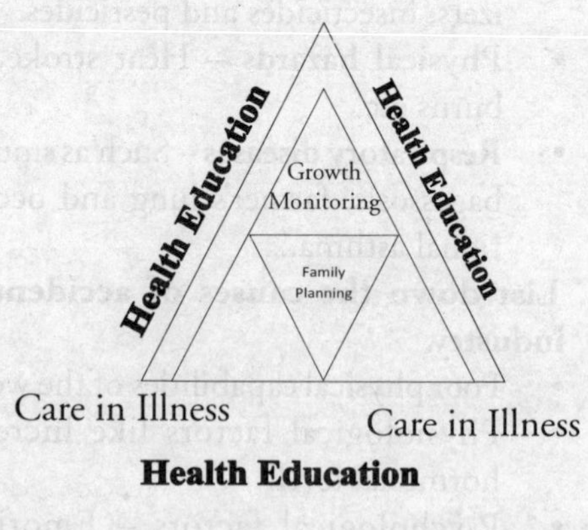

Test Series IV

1. **Mention the functions of UNICEF.**
   - Child survival growth and development.
   - Protective and learning environment.
   - Adolescent empowerment
   - Evidence based policy influencing & advocacy
2. **List down the qualities of ASHA.**
   - A woman (Married/widow/divorced).
   - Age group of 25-45 years.
   - Resident of same village.
   - Completed 8th standard of formal education.
   - Should have good communication and leadership skills.
3. **List down advantages of rapid sand filter.**
   - It can deal with raw water directly.
   - No preliminary storage is needed.
   - The filter bed occupy less space.
   - Filtration is rapid (40-50 time of a slow sand filter).
   - The washing of the filter is easy.
   - More flexibility in operation.
4. **Mention the different aspects of drinking water quality recommended by WHO.**
   - Acceptability aspects.
   - Microbiological aspects.
   - Chemical aspects.
   - Radiological aspects.
5. **What are complication of chicken pox.**
   Haemorrhage, pneumonia, encephalitis, acute cerebellar ataxia, Rey's syndrome in pregnancy – foetal wastage, birth defects.
6. **List down the stages of chicken pox.**
   - **Pre-eruptive stage** – Mild fever, pain in back, shivering, malaise, rashes.
   - **Eruptive stage** – Distribution of rash rapid evolution, pleomorphism and fever.
7. **Define measles.**
   It is an acute infectious disease of childhood caused by a specific virus called myxovirus. It is clinically characterized by fever and catarrhal symptoms of upper respiratory tract infections, followed by typical rash.
8. **Define whooping cough.**
   It is an acute infectious disease, usually of young children caused by B. pertusis. It is clinically characterized by an insidious onset with mild fever and irritating cough, gradually becoming paroxysmal with the characteristic whoop. The Chinese call it as 100 day cough.
9. **Define Ventilation.**
   Ventilation means the constant replacement of foul air by supply of fresh outdoor air with control of quality of temperature humidity and purity of the incoming air.

10. Mention the better foods at low costs.

- Plant foods high in protein like – Beans, peas, lentils, groundnuts.
- Dark green leafy vegetables.
- Main food such as – Wheat, rice or maize, ragi, raddish.

11. Define health care.

"Multitude of services rendered to individuals, families and communities by the agents of health services or professionals for the purpose of promoting, maintaining or restoring health.

12. List components of health system.

- Concepts (e.g.: Health and disease).
- Ideas (e.g.: Equity, effectiveness, efficacy).
- Objects (e.g.: Hospitals, health centres, health programme).
- Persons (e.g.: Providers & consumers).
- All the components interact to support or control one another.

13. Mention the levels of prevention.

- Primordial
- Primary
- Secondary
- Tertiary

14. Define epidemic.

An epidemic is defined as the occurrence of a disease in an area – clearly in excess of the normal expectations, e.g.: Sudden outbreak of disease.

15. Define endemic.

An endemic is defined as the occurrence of a disease round the year in a population in habituating a geographic area. The disease agent is constantly present in the endemic area and not imported from outside.

16. Define sporadic.

Sporadic is defined as the occurrence of a disease in a scattered form, independently irregularly and haphazardly, showing no common source or mutual connection e.g.: Plague.

17. List the indications for medical termination of pregnancy.

- Sound medical reason.
- Eugenic.
- Social reason.
- Humanitarian.
- Failure of contraceptives.

18. List down the dietary impact upon health.

- Consumption of poor calcium diet cause osteoporosis.
- Intake of high salty diet cause hypertension.
- Intake of alcohol induce pharyngeal, oesophageal cancer, cirrhosis of liver.
- Consumption of affluent diet cause – Hypertension, coronary heart disease and diabetes.

19. List down the objectives of antenatal care.

- To maintain the health and wellbeing of pregnant women and their fetuses.
- To identify risk factors and apply the appropriate measures of intervention as early as possible.
- To identify the complications of pregnancy'. Institute immediate remedial measures.
- To impart health education to women on pregnancy and child birth.
- To lay the foundations of a healthy pregnancy outcome and good mother child relationship.

20. Name barrier methods of contraceptives.

- Condom (Male & Female).
- Vaginal sponge.
- Diaphragm.
- Chemical forms like creams, foams, jelly's and suppositories.

21. List the advantages of home visit.

- Permits the community health nurse to observe and analyze the home and family situation in action.
- To gain confidence by personalized contact.
- To observe actual care given by family members.

22. Define family planning.

It is defined as "A way of thinking and living that is adopted voluntarily upon the basis of knowledge, attitudes and responsible decisions by individuals and couples, in order to promote the health and welfare of the family group and thus contribute effectively to the social development of a country".

23. List down objectives of family planning.

- To avoid unwanted births.
- To bring about wanted births
- To regulate the intervals between pregnancies
- To determine the number of children in the family

24. Define congenital disorder?

Congenital disorders are defined as "those diseases that are substantially determined before or during birth and which are in principle recognizable in early life".

25. List down the causes of congenital malformation.

- Genetic factors like 1) chromosomal abnormalities 2) Inborn errors of metabolism 3) Other chromosomal single gene disorders.
- Intrauterine infections such as rubella, cytomegalovirus, toxoplasmosis, syphilis.
- Maternal diseases e.g.: Diabetes mellitus, cardiac failure
- Dietary factor e.g.: Folic deficiency.

26. List down objective of school health services.

- The promotion of positive health
- The prevention of diseases
- Early diagnosis, treatment and follow up of defects
- Awakening health consciousness in children
- The promotion of healthful environment

27. Define handicap.

It may be defined as "reduction in a person's capacity to fulfill a social role as a consequence of an impairment, inadequate training for the role, or other circumstances. Applied to children the term usually refers to the presence of an impairment or other circumstances that are likely to interfere with normal growth and development or with the capacity to learn".

28. List down the principles of accident promotion in an industry.

- Adequate pre placement examination.
- Adequate job training.
- Continuing education.
- Ensuring safe working environment.
- Establishing a safety department in the organization.
- Periodic survey to find out hazards.
- Careful reporting, maintenance of records and publicity.

29. List down the benefits for employees under ESI Act.

- Medical benefit
- Sickness benefit
- Maternity benefits
- Disablement benefit
- Dependent's benefit
- Funeral expenses
- Rehabilitation allowance

30. What is ionizing radiation?
It is the radiation which has the ability to penetrate tissues and deposit its energy.

31. List down the types of ionized radiation.
- **Electromagnetic radiation** – X rays and gamma rays.
- **Corpuscular radiation** – Alpha particles, electrons

32. Mention the diseases transmitted through human excreta.
- Typhoid
- Paratyphoid
- Cholera, gastroenteritis
- Viral hepatitis
- Ascariasis
- Hook worm disease
- Poliomyelitis etc.

33. List down the qualities of suitable latrine.
- It should be acceptable to people.
- It should be simple in constitution.
- It should be simple to use.
- It should be cheap and materials for construction and it should be locally available.
- It should involve the use of very small amount of water.
- It should be hygiene and sanitary.
- It should not lead to environmental pollution.

34. Mention the two signs of successful breast feeding.
- Alert appearance of the baby.
- Normal tissue turgor.
- At least 5 wet nappies day.
- Adequate weight gain.

35. How many days colostrum is secreted?
First 2-3 days after delivery.

36. Enlist the uses of vital statistics.
- To find out the leading causes of morbidity and mortality.
- To promote health legislation.
- To evaluate the governmental health programme (success or failure).
- To discover solution for health problems.
- To estimate future need.
- For planning and administration of health series.
- To direct, maintain and control during execution of program.
- For production of health trends.
- For prioritizing the health programmes.

37. Name methods or sources of vital statistics.
- Population Census.
- Civil Registration System.
- Sample Registration System.
- Medical certification causes of death.
- Community survey.
- National sample survey.
- Model registration system.
- Hospital records.
- Epidemiological surveillance report.

38. What are the problems faced by urban slum population in India.
- Health Problems: Diarrhoea, sexually transmitted disease, skin infections, malignancy.
- Environmental Problems: Atmospheric pollution (Air, water, soil pollutions, road accidents).
- Economic Problems: Poverty.
- Social Problems: Alcoholism, drug abuse, prostitution.
- Psychological Problem: Anxiety, stress, suicide.

39. List down the changes in Indian family.
- Loosening of social regulation.
- Indian women behaves like western culture.

- Face difficulty in reproductive and child health period.
- Deteriorating kinship in the family.
- Divorce rate is increasing.
- Diversity in family norms.

40. Name few child welfare agencies in India.
- Indian Council for Child Welfare (I.C.C.W).
- Central Social Welfare Board.
- Kasturba Memorial Trusts.
- Indian Red Cross Society.

41. Name diseases with which Siddha is very effective.
- Chronic liver diseases.
- Skin diseases like psoriasis.
- Rheumatic problem.
- Anaemia.
- Prostate enlargement.
- Bleeding piles and peptic ulcer.

42. Define human migration.

Human migration is movement by humans from one district to another sometimes over long distances in large groups.

43. Define community organization.

"Community organization is a process by which the community is able to identify its needs and take actions to fulfill their needs or solve the problems" – Murray and Gross.

44. Mention the categories of CAM.
- Alternative medical system.
- Body mind intervention.
- Biological based therapy.
- Manipulation and body based method
- Energy therapy.

45. How many home visits should be provided for every newborn baby by a health worker according to IMNCI Protocol?

There are three home visits

1st visit – On the day of birth (First day)
2nd visit – On the 3rd day
3rd visit – On the 7th day

For low birth weight babies, 3 more visits are to be undertaken before the baby is one month of age.

46. List down the viruses causing diarrhoea.
- Rota viruses
- Astro viruses
- Corona viruses
- Adeno viruses
- Norwalk group viruses
- Calci viruses
- Entero viruses

47. Name bacteria causing diarrhoea.
- Escherichia coli
- Shigella
- Vibrio cholerae
- Campylo bacter jejuni
- Solmonella

48. Name the toxin present in khesari dal which causes neurolathyrism.

The toxin present in Lathyrus seeds has been identified as beta oxalyl amino alanine (BOAA). Studies indicate that there is a blood brain barrier to this toxin.

49. How will you remove the toxin (BOAA) from khesari dal?

Removing the toxin from the pulse by soaking it in hot water and rejecting the soaked water.

50. List down few methods of pasteurization of milk.

Holder (Vat) Method
- **Milk kept at 63 – 66°C for 30 mins** quickly cooled to 5°C.
- **HTST Method** – High temperature and short time method.
- Milk heated to 72°C, held at 15 seconds rapidly cooled to 4°C.
- **UHT Method** – Ultra high tempera ture method

Test Series V

1. **Define ARI.**
   It refers to Acute Respiratory Infection and it is acute infectious disease and it may cause inflammation of the respiratory tract anywhere from nose to alveoli with a range of combination of signs and symptoms.
2. **List down the signs and symptoms of dry malnutrition or marasmus.**
   Not eating enough food, an old man face, always hungry, pot belly, very thin, underweight. The child is just like skin and bones.
3. **List down the signs and symptoms of wet malnutrition or kwashiorkor.**
   Not eating enough protein, swollen moon face, stopped growing, color loss in hair and skin, thin upper arms, sores and peeling skin, swollen hands and feet, wasted muscles. The child is skin bones and water.
4. **List down the typical signs of anaemia.**
   - Pale or transparent skin.
   - Shiny smooth tongue.
   - Paleness insides of eyelids.
   - White fingernails.
   - Pale gums
   - Weakness and
   - Fatigue
5. **Mention +ive reaction of Mantoux test.**
   After administration of PPD 0.1 ml intradermally in left forearm waiting for 72 hours. The reaction occurs. The reaction consists of erythema and induration. The reaction exceeding 10mm are considered as "positive reaction".
6. **Define disinfectant.**
   A disinfectant or germicide is a substance which destroys harmful microbes (not usually spores) with the aim of preventing transmission of disease.
7. **List down types of disinfectants.**
   - Physical – Burning, hot air, boiling, autoclaving radiation.
   - Natural – Sunlight, Air.
   - Chemical – Phenol, ammonia, halogens, alcohols, formaldehyde etc.
8. **List down the divisions of health sector in India.**
   - Water supply and sanitation.
   - Control of communicable diseases.
   - Medical education, training and research.
   - Medical care including hospitals, dispensaries and primary health centres.
   - Public health services.
   - Family planning.
   - Indigenous systems of medicine.

9. List down the 18 highly focused states under NRHM.

Bihar, Jharkhand, Madhya Pradesh, Chattisgarh, Uttar Pradesh, Uttaranchal, Orissa, Rajasthan, Assam, Arunachal Pradesh, Manipur, Meghalaya, Mizoram, Nagaland, Sikkim, Tripura, Himachal Pradesh, Jammu and Kashmir.

10. List down the health impact of improper waste management.

- Nuisance from bad odours.
- Water and soil pollution.
- Breeding place of flies and mosquitoes.
- It attracts rodents and vermin.
- Spread of communicable diseases.

11. List down the types of latrine.

1. Service type latrine.
2. Non service type latrine.

- Bore hole latrine.
- Dug well latrine.
- Water seal latrine.
- RCA latrine.
- Sulabh community latrines.
- Shallow trench latrine.
- Deep trench latrine.

12. Define sewage.

Sewage is a waste water from a community containing solid and liquid excreta, derived from houses, street and yard washings, factories and industries. It resembles dirty water with unpleasant smell.

13. How the diseases can be classified?

Diseases can be classified on the basis of

- Aetiological agents.
- Pathological changes.
- Clinical manifestations.
- Organ system involvement or epidemiological characteristics.

14. List down the four important generator of mosquito transmit diseases.

- Anopheles
- Culex
- Ades
- Mansonia

15. Mention the 2 larvivorus fish for devouring the cyclops.

- Barbal fish
- Gambasia fish

16. Who are responsible for health care?

- Individual responsibility.
- Community responsibility.
- State responsibility.
- International responsibility.

17. List down the aspects of family planning.

- Women's Health – To prevent maternal mortality and morbidity of woman, adequate nutritional status prevent complication of pregnancy and abortion.
- Foetal Health – To prevent foetal mortality and abnormal development.
- Infant & child health – To prevent neonatal, infant and preschool mortality, vulnerability to diseases etc.

18. List down the scope of family planning.

- Proper spacing and limitation of birth.
- Advice on sterility.
- Education for parenthood.
- Sex education.
- Screening of diseases (e.g.,: cervical cancers).
- Genetic counseling.
- Premarital consultation and examination.
- To carry out pregnancy tests.
- Manage counseling.
- Preparation of couples to receive their first child.
- Services to unmarried mothers.
- Providing adoption services.

19. Define couple protection rate.

It is defined as the rate of eligible couples effectively protected against child birth by one or the other approved methods of family planning viz. sterilization, IUD, Condom, oral Pills etc.

20. What is the two different basic types of Intrauterine Device?

- Non medicated
- Medicated

21. What is the ideal time of intrauterine device insertion?

During menstruation or within 10 days of menstrual period.

22. Define disability.

It is defined as "any restriction or lack of ability to perform an activity in a manner or within the range considered normal for a human being". Impairment leads to disability.

23. Define impairment.

It is defined as "any loss or abnormality of psychological, physiological or anatomical structure or function".

24. How will you classify handicapped children?

- Physically handicapped.
- Mentally handicapped.
- Socially handicapped.

25. Classify behaviour problems in children.

- **Problems antisocial in nature** – E.g. Stealing, lying, gambling, cruelty, etc.
- **Habit disorders** – E.g. Nail biting, thumb sucking, bed wetting and masturbation.
- **Personality disorders** – E.g. Temper tantrums, jealousy, shyness, day dreaming, fears and anxiety
- **Psychosomatic complaints** – E.g. Tremors, headache, asthma, delusion, hallucination, etc.
- **Educational difficulties** – E.g. School phobia, school failure, backwardness in studies.

26. What are the health hazards faced by slum dwellers?

- **Respiratory Infections** – Common cold, TB, Influenza.
- **Rat infestation** – Plague.
- **Arthropod nuisance** – Housefly, mosquito, fleas bugs.
- **Accidents** – Fire, etc.
- **Psychosocial effects** – Insecurity feeling, isolation, delinquency and drug abuse etc.

27. Give few examples of sanitary latrines.

- Bore hole latrine.
- Dug well latrine.
- Water seal latrine – RCA type.
- Chemical closet.
- Septic tank.

28. List down the environment hazards due to industrialization.

- **Substandard housing** – Emergence of slums.
- **Water pollution** –Mixing of acid alkalis oil in the drinking water.
- **Air pollution** – Toxic gases fumes dusts to the atmospheric air.
- **Improper sewage disposal** – Communicable disease transmission, water pollution, skin infection etc.

29. Name the sexually transmitted diseases.

- **Syphilis** – Treponema pallidum.
- **Gonorrhoea** – Neisseria gonorrhea.
- **Chancroid** – Haemophilus ducreyi
- **Lympho granuloma venereum** – Chlamydia trachomatis.
- **Granuloma inguinale** – Calymmato bacterium granulomatis.
- Non-specific urethritis.

- AIDS – HIV virus.

30. List down the method of rehabilitation for blindness.

- **Physical rehabilitation** – Establishment of eye banks
- **Social rehabilitation** – Special schools and homes for rehabilitation
- **Vocational rehabilitation** – Providing gainful employment
- **Psychological rehabilitation** – Giving psychological support

31. List down the problems requiring urgent attention in India.

- Nutrition-Adequate nutrition for whole population
- Prevention of food adulteration
- Water supply and sanitation
- Environmental protection
- Immunization programme
- MCH services
- School health programmes
- Occupational health services

32. How will you calculate volume of water in the well?

D – Diameter of well in meter

H – Depth of water column in meter

2.5 gm of good quality bleaching powder to disinfect 1000 litres of water

33. List the effects of noise.

- **Auditory effect** – Auditory fatigue deafness.
- **Non auditory** – Speech interference, annoyance, decreased efficacy.
- **Physiological changes** – Increased BP, increased heart rate, increased sweating, giddiness, nausea, fatigue, insomnia, visual disturbance.

34. List down high temperature induced disorders.

- Heat stroke
- Heat exhaustion
- Heat cramps
- Heat syncope
- Heat rash
- Others – Complaints of discomfort, irritability, lassitude, anxiety, lowered morale and lack of concentration.

35. List down the dust induced diseases.

They are called pneumoconiosis (chronic pulmonary fibrosis of restrictive type)

- Silicosis (Localised nodular type)
- Byssinosis (Brown lung)
- Bagassosis
- Siderosis
- Asbestosis
- Anthracosia
- Tabaccosis
- Farmer's lung

36. Define colustrum.

Colostrum is the major secretion of breast during the first week of lactation.

37. Mention the positioning of the newborn while breast feeding.

- Cradle hold position
- Football hold
- Side lying

38. What is a self help group?

It is a group of 12 to 20 women belonging to the lower economic class who come forward voluntarily to work together for their own economic uplift.

39. Name legislations upon child health.

- The Child labour Act – 1986.
- Child marriage restraint Act – 1978.
- The Children act – 1960 (Mainly for neglected and destitute, delinquent children).
- Juvenile justice act – 1986.

40. List down the few method of treatment or the therapies under naturopathy.

- Water therapy
- Food therapy
- Air therapy
- Massage therapy
- Fire therapy
- Acupressure
- Mud therapy
- Magnetic therapy
- Chromatherapy (VIBGYOR)
- Music and Art therapy
- Acupuncture
- Animal assisted therapy e.g.,: leech therapy
- Meditation
- Biological based therapies like
- Herbal therapy
- Aromatherapy
- Nutritional therapy
- YOGA
- Energy therapies like therapeutic touch, reiki, magnet therapy etc.

41. List down the types of human migration.

- Voluntary migration.
- Involuntary migration.

42. Define Gross Reproductive Rate (GRR).

GRR = Average number of children that would be born to married woman on experiencing the current fertility pattern throughout her reproductive span.

43. Define Net Reproductive Rate (NRR).

NRR = Number of daughters a new born girl will bear during her lifetime assuming fixed age specific fertility, mortality rates. Current Net Reproduction Rate is 1.

44. What is Crude Marriage Rate?

$$CMR = \frac{\text{No. of marriages in the year}}{\text{Mild year population}} \times 1000$$

45. Define Couple Protection Rate.

CPR = Percentage of eligible couples effectively protected against contraception by one or the other approved methods of contraception (fertility regulation).

46. List down the components of school health programme.

- School Health Service – Including health appraisal, immunization, emergency care, care of common illness, maintaining hygiene etc.
- Health promoting school environment.
- Physical facilities.
- Play and recreation.
- Prevention of accidents and injuries.
- Consultation with school authorities.
- School health curriculum – should aim to bring out desirable changes in health knowledge attitude and practice.

47. List three principles used in homeopathy.

- Law of similar • Law of single remedy
- Law of minimum dose

48. List down the various tests to check the efficiency of milk pasteurization.

- Phosphatase test • Standard plate count
- Coliform count

49. When did balwadi nutrition programme launched and what is the amount of food supplement?

The programme was started in 1970 for the benefit of children in the age group 3-6 years in rural areas.

The food supplement provides 300 Kcal and 10 grams of protein per child per day.

50. What is the other name of mid day meal scheme?

Mid day meal scheme is also known as national programme of nutritional support to primary education.

Test Series VI

1. **When did the WHO declare small pox completely eradicated from the entire world?**
In the WHO Assembly of May 8, 1980
2. **Mention the panchayat raj at village level.**
The Gram Sabha: Assembly of all the adults in the village. They meet at least twice in a year.
Gram Panchayat: It is the executive organ of the gram sabha and an agency for planning and development at the village level.
The Niyaya Panchayat: They cover the entire field of our administration.
3. **Define planning commission.**
Planning commission are formulated to make an assessment of the material, capital and human resources of the country and to draft developmental plans for the most effective utilization of these resources.
4. **Mention the composition of sewage.**
Sewage contains 99.9 percent of water 0.1 percent of the solids which are partly organic and partly inorganic and partly in suspension and partly in solution.
5. **List down the habits of mosquitoes.**
    - Feeding habits
    - Biting habits
    - Resting habits
    - Breeding habits
    - Hibernation
    - Disposal
6. **Mention the biological control of mosquito larvae.**
Small fish feed readily on mosquito larvae
    - Gambusia affinis (Gambusia fish)
    - Lebistes reticulatus (Barbal fish)
7. **List down the habits of housefly.**
    - Breeding habits
    - Feeding habits
    - Restlessness
    - Vomit drop habit
    - Defecation
    - Resting habits
    - Disposal
8. **What are all the ways flies transmit diseases?**
    - Mechanical transmission
    - Vomit drop & through defecations
9. **List down most common disease spreading fleas in India.**
    1. **Rat fleas** – Xenopsylla cheopis (Oriental) Xenopsylla astia Xenopsylla braziliensis
    2. **Rat fleas** – Nosopsylla fasciatus (Temperate zone)
    3. **Human fleas** – Pulex Gritans

4. **Dog and cat fleas** – Etonocephalus canis Etonocephalus felis
5. **Sand fleas** – Tunga penetrans

10. What disease itch mite cause and when did they discovered?

Itchmite causes a disease called Scabies (Sarcoptes scabei or acarus scabies). They discovered in 1687

11. List down the lice causing disease in human being.

- Epidemic typhus
- Relapsing fever
- Trench fever
- Dermatitis

12. Define contamination.

It is defined as the presence of an infectious agent on the body surface also on or in the clothes, beddings, toys, surgical instruments or dressing and other inanimate articles or substances including water, milk and food.

13. Who is ideal Intrauterine Device candidate by PPFAC (Planned Parenthood Federation of America)?

- Who has at least one child
- Who has no history of pelvic disease
- Who has normal menstrual periods
- Who is willing to check the Intrauterine Device tail
- Who has access to follow up and treatment of potential problems
- Who is having a monogamous relationship

14. Name types of oral pills.

- Combined pill
- Progesterone only pill
- Post coital pill
- Once a month pill

5. Male pill

15. What is coitus interruptus?

This is the oldest method of voluntary fertility control. It involves no cost or appliances. The male withdraws before ejaculation, and thereby tries to prevent deposition of semen into the vagina.

16. What is immunization in family planning?

Immunization with HCG (Human Chronic Gonadotropin) which could block continuation of pregnancy. Antibodies appeared in about 4 – 6 weeks and the immunity period ranging from 6 – 11 months. Then the immunity can be boosted by second injection.

17. What are all the psychological problems of man after male sterilization?

- Diminution of sexual vigor
- Feeling of impotence
- Headache, fatigue

18. List down the objectives of ICDSs scheme.

- To improve the nutritional and health status of children in the age group 0-6 years.
- To lay the foundations for proper psychological, physical and social development of the child.
- To reduce mortality and morbidity, malnutrition and school drop out.
- To achieve an effective coordination of policy and implementation among various departments for promoting child development.
- To enhance the capability of the mother and nutritional needs of the child through proper nutrition and health education.

19. What are the services rendered by ICDS for pregnant women.

- Health checkup
- Immunization (Injection T.T)
- Supplementary nutrition

- Nutrition and health education

20. List down the services rendered by ICDS for 3-6 years children.

- Supplementary nutrition
- Immunization
- Health checkup
- Referral services
- Non formal education

21. List down the signs of vitamin A deficiency.

- Night blindness
- Conjunctival xerosis
- Bitot's Spots
- Corneal xerosis
- Keratomalacia
- Xeropthalmia

22. List down the prevention and control of human plague.

I. Control of Cases

- Notification isolation
- Treatment

II. Control of Fleas

- Coincide with anti-rodent measures
- Dusting of DDT and BHC
- Disinfection

III. Control of rodents – Mass destruction

IV. Vaccination

V. Chemoprophylaxis

VI. Surveillance

VII. Health education

23. List down the types of tetanus.

- **Traumatic**–Trauma
- **Puerperal** – Abortion
- **Otogenic – Infected foreign bodies**
  Idiopathic – Microscopic trauma
- **Tetanus Neonatrum** – Infection of umbilical stump after birth

24. List down five tenets of DOTs.

- Political commitment for tuberculosis control.
- Detection of tuberculosis cases by sputum smear microscopy. Those who attend health care facility with the complaints of cough for more than 3 weeks.
- Standard treatment regimens for 6-8 months with direct observation for at least first month.
- Regular and uninterrupted supply of anti-tuberculosis drugs.
- Systemic monitoring and accountability for each patient of tuberculosis.

25. List down the occupational disorders.

- Noise induced disorders
- Occupational dermatitis
- Industrial accidents
- Vibration induced disorder
- Ionising rotation induced disorders
- Dust induced disorders
- Chronic lead poisoning
- Stress induced disorders

26. List important arthropod borne diseases.

- **Mosquito** – Malaria, filariasis, yellow fever, dengue etc.
- **Housefly** – Enteric fever, diarrhoea, dysentery, cholera, gastro enteritis, polio
- **Sandfly** – Kala azar, oriental sore, sandfly fever
- **Tsetsefly** – Sleeping sickness
- **Louse** – Epidemic typhus, relapsing fever, trench fever
- **Ratfleas** – Bubonic plague, endemic typhus etc.
- **Blackfly** – Onchoceriasis
- **Reduviid bug** – Chaga's disease
- **Hard tick** – Tick typhus, viral encephalitis, tularemia etc.
- **Soft tick** – Relapsing fever
- **Trombiculid mite** – Scrub typhus
- **Itchmite** – Scabies

- Cyclops – Guinea

27. List important social security acts available in India.
- The Factories Act, 1976
- The Employee State Insurance Act, 1975
- The Mines Act
- The Plantation Act
- The Minimum Wages Act
- The Maternity Benefit Act

28. List down few occupational dermatitis.
- Arsenic keratosis
- Baker's dermatitis
- Asbestos corns
- Beryllium granuloma
- Oil acne
- Chromate dermatitis
- Chlor acne
- Dhobi itch, etc.

29. What is predominant breast feeding?

Breast feeding a baby along with small amount of water or water based drinks.

30. Define transitional milk.

It appears as the milk, when the milk changes from colostrum to mature milk.

31. List down the functions of SHGs.

Empower women by various progammes such as income generation leading to credit repayment, marketing savings internal rotation of money, maintaining accounts

Establish linkages with banks and other institution

Participate in village level social development activities

Act as agents of change

32. Explain social importance of customs.
- Regulates social behaviour
- Moulds personality of the individual
- Custom preserves the culture
- Custom transmits the culture to succeeding generations
- It supports laws, provides solid grounds for the formulation and establishment of laws
- It is demonstration and totalitarian of self expression

33. Define marriage.

Marriage is a socially approved relation which allows sexual relationship between two individuals of opposite sex.

34. Explain importance of marriage.
- Regulates sex life and sex relation of the individual
- Puts restrictions on the premarital and extra marital sex relations
- Marriage develops intense love and affection towards each other
- Marriage helps intellectual cooperation among both the spouses
- Minimizes the social distance between groups and strengthen their solidarity

35. Define Family.

Family is the biological social unit is composed of husband, wife and children

36. List various health problems in childhood period.
- Low birth weight
- Protein energy malnutrition
- Micro nutrient malnutrition. E.g. : Vitamin A, calcium, iron, zinc, iodine
- Accidents
- Nutritional Anaemia
- Nutritional blindness
- Infections
- Poisoning
- Behavioural problems

37. What is the impact of human migration.
- Increases urbanization
- Increases industrialization
- Cultural change

- Civilization
- Economic recession
- Sometime conflict and climatic change
- Changes in population distribution
- Cultural spread throughout world

38. Name the measurements in community health.

- Measurement of mortality. E.g. IMR, MMR, NMR, U5MR etc.
- Measurement of morbidity of incidence and prevalence of disease conditions
- Measurement of disability. E.g. Disability adjusted life years (DALY)
- Measurement of natality – E.g. Birth rate
- Measurements of presence/absence or distribution of the characteristics of the disease
- Measurement of health care needs
- Measurement of demographic variables
- Measurement of the presence/absence of distribution of environmental or health related events

39. List down the tools and measurement in community.

Rates: Is obtained by the number of persons diagnosed as sick with the number of people examined multiplied with a standard value. E.g.: Death rate

$$\frac{\text{Number of Deaths in year}}{\text{Mild year population}} \times 1000$$

Ratio: Expresses a relation in size between the random quantities. The numerator is not a component of the denominator.

e.g., X: Y or X/Y

No. of Male: No. of Females

Proportion: Is ratio that indicates the relation in magnitude of a part of the whole.

$$\frac{\text{No. of children with diarrhoea in a village}}{\text{Total no. of children of the same village}} \times 1000$$

40. List down various health indicators.

- Morbidity indicator
- Mortality indicator
- Disability rate
- Nutritional status indicator
- Health care delivery indicator
- Utilization rates
- Indicator of sound mental health
- Environmental indicators
- Health policy indicator
- Quality of life indicator
- Others

41. List the elements of primary health care.

E – Ensure safe water supply

L – Locally endemic disease control

E – Education & expanded programme of immunization

M – Maternal and child health including family planning

E – Environmental sanitation

N – Nutritional services & promotion of food supply

T – Treatment of common diseases and injury

S – School health services and provision of essential drugs

42. List down the three tier system of health care.

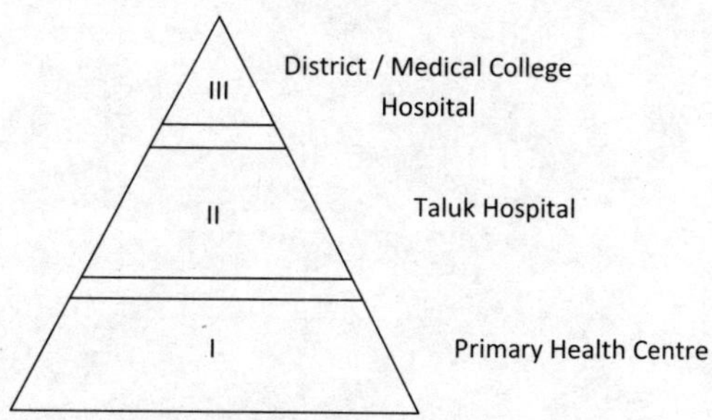

43. List down few characteristics of indigenous systems of medicine.

- The ISM practitioner treats the whole patient rather than the diseases structure/organ/system.
- The ISM diagnosis and treatment are individualized. No two patients receive the same treatment even if they have same clinical features.
- A spiritual element is often incorporated in ISM therapies.

44. Mention colours used in chromotherapy.

Called VIBGYOR, alphabets stand for

V - Violet
I - Indigo
B - Blue
G - Green
Y - Yellow
O - Orange
R - Red

45. What is the other name of mid day meal programme and when was it operated?

MDMP is also known as school lunch programme. It has been in operation since 1961 throughout the country.

46. Name the unit of measurement of loudness of noise?

Sound pressure levels therefore it is expressed in dB (decibels).

47. Which are the compounds responsible for the hardness of water?

- Calcium bicarbonate
- Magnesium bicarbonate
- Calcium sulphate
- Magnesium sulphate

Carbonate hardness is temporary hardness due to presence of calcium and magnesium bicarbonates. The non-carbonate hardness is permanent hardness which is mainly due to presence of calcium and magnesium sulphates, chlorides and nitrates.

48. How does boiling removes the temporary hardness?

It is removing temporary hardness mainly by expelling carbon dioxide and precipitating the insoluble calcium carbonate.

$Ca(HCO3)2 \longrightarrow CaCO3 + H2O + CO2$

49. What is the other name of Bhore Committee, 1946?

It is Health Survey and Development Committee.

50. What is the other name of Mudaliar Committee, 1962?

It is Health Survey and Planning Committee.

Test Series VII

1. **List down the child welfare programmes in India.**
   - Midday meal programme 1961
   - Special nutrition programme 1970
   - ICDS programme 1975
   - EPI programme for immunization-1978
   - Universal immunization programme 1985
   - Under five clinic
   - CSSM programme 1992
   - Baby friendly hospital (BFH) 1993
   - RCH package I -1997
   - RCH package II -2007
   - IMNCI
2. **Mention the components of diarrhoeal disease control program.**

   In short term – Appropriate clinical management

   In long term – Better MCH care practices, preventive strategies, preventing diarrhoeal epidemics.
3. **List down the different types of hepatitis.**
   - Hepatitis A
   - Hepatitis B
   - Hepatitis C
   - Hepatitis D
   - Hepatitis E
   - Hepatitis F
   - Hepatitis G
4. **List down the components of filarial survey.**
   - Mass blood survey
   - Clinical survey
   - Serological tests
   - Xerodiagnosis
   - Entomological survey
5. **Define influenza.**

   It is an acute respiratory tract infection caused by influenza viruses of 3 types which are A, B and E. All known pandemic were caused by influenza A strains. The disease characterized by sudden onset of chills, malaise, fever and muscular pain and cough.
6. **Define nosocomial infection.**

   Nosocomial infection originating in a patient while in a hospital or other health care facility. It denotes a new disorder associated with being in a hospital.
7. **Define contamination.**

   It is defined as the presence of an infectious agent on the body surface also on or in the clothes, beddings, toys, surgical instruments or dressing and other inanimate articles or substance including water milk and food.
8. **Define communicable period.**

   It is defined as "the time during which an infectious agent may be transferred directly or indirectly from the infected person to another person, which may from an infected animal to man or infected man to animal including arthropods".

9. Define external environment/macro environment.

It is defined as "all that which is external to the individual human host". It can be physical, biological and psychosocial components any or all which can affect the health of man.

10. List down the health care delivery indicators.

Doctors-population ratio, Doctor-Nurse rates, population bed ratio, population per health/subcentre, population per traditional birth attendant.

11. List down the kinds of thermometers used for measuring temperature of air?

- Ordinary mercury thermometer
- Maximum thermometer (It has either an iron index above mercury column).
- Minimum thermometer (Alcohol filled).
- Six's thermometer (U shaped glass body bent thermometer).
- Globe Thermometer.
- Wet Globe Thermometer.

12. List the types of instruments available for measuring humidity.

- Dry and wet bulb thermometers.
- Sling psychometer or whirling psychometer.
- Assmann psychometer.

13. List down the intrauterine hormonal devices of 3rd generation pills.

Progestasert, Levonorgestrel

14. Define passive immunization.

It is a process of conferring immunity by administering readymade antibodies of human or animal origin. The immunity offers specific protection for a limited period lasting for a few months and useful for short term prophylaxis.

15. List down various method of disease transmission.

- Contact borne
- Air borne
- Vehicle borne
- Fomite borne
- Vector borne
- Vertical borne e.g.: mother to foetus
- Hand borne transmission (Finger) 5F's

16. What is innate immunity?

It is passed on from the mother to offspring. It is non-specific and broad based not detect against any infective agent.

17. What do you mean by incubation period?

In all communicable diseases, a period of time interval between the occurrence of infection and the appearance of the first clinical manifestations. This interval time is called incubation period.

18. Mention the two methods of conducting female sterilization.

- Laparoscopy
- Mini laparotomy

19. List down the stages of maternity cycle.

- Fertilization
- Antenatal or prenatal period
- Intra natal period
- Postnatal period
- Inter conceptional period

20. List down the maternal and child health problems in India.

- **Malnutrition** – Pregnant women, nursing mothers and children by low birth weight babies, anemia, toxemias of pregnancy, postpartum haemorrhage lead to high mortality rate.

- **Infection** – Maternal infection leads to foetal growth retardation, low birth weight babies embryopathy, abortion and puerperal sepsis, cytomegalo viruses, herpes simplex or toxoplasma during pregnancy, TORCH infection and infectious disease during pregnancy. E.g., TB, HIV/AIDS
- **Uncontrolled reproduction** – Leads to high maternal and perinatal mortality.

21. What do you mean by minimum 3 visits of antenatal mother?

1st visit at 20 weeks or as soon as pregnancy occurs

2nd visit at 32 weeks

3rd visit at 36 weeks

22. Who are all high risk antenatal mothers?

- Elderly primi (30 years and above)
- Short (statured primi-140 cm and below)
- Malpresentations viz, breech, transcience etc.
- Antepartum haemorrhage, threatened abortion
- Preeclampsia and eclampsia
- Anaemia
- Twins, hydramnios
- Previous still birth, intrauterine death
- Elderly grand multi paras
- Prolonged pregnancy (14 days after expected date of delivery)
- Pregnancy associated with general diseases e.g., IUD, Diabetes Mellitus, Tuberculosis, Liver disease etc.

23. What is Gomez classification?

Gomez classification is based on weight retardation. It locates the child on the basis of his or her weight in comparison with a normal child of same age.

Weight for age % =

$$\frac{\text{Weight of the child}}{\text{Weight of a normal child same age}} \times 100$$

Between 90 and 110% : Normal nutritional status

Between 75 and 89% : 1st degree malnutrition

Between 60 and 74% : 2nd degree moderate malnutrition

Under 60% : 3rd degree severe malnutrition

24. Define nutritional anaemia.

It is defined as "a condition in which the haemoglobin content of blood is lower than normal as a result of a deficiency of one or more essential nutrients regardless of the cause of such deficiency – WHO.

25. Define dental fluorosis.

Fluorosis of dental enamel occurs when excess fluoride is ingested during the years of tooth calcification, during the first 7 years of life which is characterized by "Mottling" of dental enamel mainly at the levels above 1.5 mg/L intake.

26. List down the different methods of dietary survey.

- Weighing of raw foods
- Weighing of cooked foods
- Questionnaire method

27. What is integrated approach for vector control?

It is the combining of two or more vector control method, whether these are directed only on the larvae or adults or both in order to obtain maximum results with the minimum effort and to avoid the excessive use of any one method.

28. List down the aims of school health service.

- To prevent diseases in school children and to promote their health, growth and development.

- To inculcate in them the correct attitudes, habits and practices regarding health, sex, family welfare and parenthood.
- To manipulate the social milieu of the school so as to assist satisfactory socialization of children.

29. List down the factors responsible for industrial accidents.

- Explosions, roof collapses
- Inundation of mines with water
- Land slides and border falls
- Fall into pits, unprotected with barricades
- Ill destroyed tools or machinery
- Non fencing and emission of flying slivers and sparks.

30. Mention the form of the carbohydrate content of the breast milk.

Lactose

31. Mention the duration of exclusive breast feeding.

Until six months of age

32. List down the participatory learning methods in community.

- Transact analysis
- Social mapping
- Seasonality diagram
- Focus group discussion
- Body mapping
- Wealth ranking
- Vein diagram

33. List down the concepts of family.

- **Biological concepts** – Biological function of family
- **Psychological concepts** – Prevention of mental illness
- **Economical concepts** – Meet their financial need
- **Sociological concepts** – It focus on dynamic internal and external relationship and family with society

34. List down the types of family.

It is classified based on different aspects.

By Dominance

Nuclear family – Elementary family of married family couple and their unmarried children

Joint family – Couple with their children's family lives together

Extended family – Husband, wife, children and their dependents like brothers, sisters stay together

By Marriage

Polygamy – One marries many women and lives in a family with his wives and children

Polyandrous – Women marries many man and lives in a family with all of them or with each of them alternatively

Monogamous – One man marries only one woman and established a family

According to Ancestry

Matrilineal – Mother is the basis of ancestry

Patrilineal – Father is the basis of ancestry

According to Residence

Matrilocal – The husband lives in the wife's home

Patrilocal – The wife lives in the husband's home

Changing residence – Husband and wife alternatively change their residence

According to Authority

Patriarchial – The father is the most powerful

Matriarchial family – Mother plays a dominant role in the family

35. List down the stages in family cycle.

- Formative
- Child bearing

- Growth stage
- Maturity stage
- Retraction stage

36. List down the basic needs of the family.

- **Physical Need** – Food, safe water, clothing, safe environment, shelter, safe disposal of waste
- **Biological need** – Free from communicable diseases, control of insects and rodents
- **Psychosocial need** – Happy home, adequate medical care, safe working environment, psycho-social security

37. List down the family problems in India.

- Dowry system
- Infertility, sterility
- Marital disharmony
- Egoism
- Conflict due to non adaptation of culture
- Broken family
- Poor social adjustment
- Economic problem
- Malnutrition, alcoholism
- Susceptibility to diseases
- Chronic illness in the family

38. List down the causes of human migration.

Causes are in push and pull factors

- Natural disasters
- Conflicts/war
- Threats to individual safety
- Poor political prospects

39. List down the essential newborn care.

- Care at birth, clean hands, clean surface, clean scissors, clean cotton, clean cord stumps.
- Provision of warmth
- Cord care
- Eye care
- Recording birth weight
- Initiation of breastfeeding

40. List down the few functions of PHC.

- Medical care
- MCH including family planning services
- Safe water supply and sanitation
- Prevention and control of locally endemic diseases
- Collection and reporting vital statistics
- Health education
- Nutritional health programmes
- Referral services
- Training of health guides, health workers, local dais and health assistants
- Basic laboratory services

41. List down the few records maintained in PHC.

- Antenatal care record
- CCR – Child Care Record about immunization
- Birth register
- Antenatal visit record
- Referral register
- Indent register

42. List down the approaches to control of infectious diseases.

- Measures aimed at destruction of the pathogen.
- Measures aimed at improving the host's resistance.
- Measures aimed at improving the efficiency of the control programme.

43. Define community health nurse.

Community health nurse is a nurse who works in a situation other than the hospital, nursing home or similar institutions. She may work in the homes, schools, industries, recreational settings or old age homes. She undergone 4 years graduate nursing course or she is a certificate/diploma holding nurse who has undergone additional training in community health nursing.

44. List down the village level health workers in community.

- Village health guide
- Anganwadi worker
- Trained birth attendant
- Skilled birth attendant
- ANM
- MPHW
- ASHA – Accredited social health activist

45. List some health NGOs in India.

- Indian Red Cross Society (IRCS)
- Tuberculosis Association of India (TAI)
- Family Planning Association of India (FPAI)
- Hind Kusht Nivaran Sangh (HKNS)
- Voluntary Health Association of India (VHAI)
- Child Relief and You (CRY)

46. Define blindness.

Blindness is defined as visual acuity of less than 3/60 (10/200) and when one cannot read letters or decibel symbols at 3m (10 feet).

47. What are child health component of RCH.

- Immunization
- Vitamin A prophylaxis
- Diarrhoea control
- Newborn baby care
- Poliomyelitis eradication
- ARI control

48. What are the two types of meditation?

- Inclusive meditation
- Exclusive meditation

49. List down few social problems in our community.

- Alcoholism
- CSW – Commercial sex worker
- Drug dependence
- Delinquency
- Sexually transmitted disease
- Dowry system

50. List down the natural resources of our country.

India is rich in natural resources and manpower resources

- Agriculture resources
- Forestry resources
- Fisheries resources
- Mineral resources
- Manpower resources

Test Series VIII

1. **Define incubation period.**
Incubation is defined as "the time interval between invasion by an infectious agent and appearance of the first sign or symptom of the disease" is called incubation Period.
2. **Define opportunistic infection.**
It is the "infection by an organism that takes the opportunity provided by a defect in the host's defense to infect the host and it causes disease. E.g.: Organism include herpes simplex, cytomegalovirus, toxoplasma, etc.
3. **Define food poisoning.**
Food poisoning is an acute gastro enteritis caused by ingestion of food or drink which also contaminated with either living bacteria or their toxins or inorganic chemical substances and poisons derived from plants and animals.
4. **Mention the types of food poisoning.**
   1. Bacterial: Ingestion of food contaminated by living bacteria or their toxins. E.g., Salmonella & staphylococcal food poisoning.
   2. Non bacteria: Ingestion of contaminated food by chemicals such as fertilizers, pesticides, cadmium, mercury, etc.
5. **Define botulism.**
It is a type of food poisoning caused by clostridium botulinum type A, B or E. The prominent symptoms of dysphagia, diplopia, ptosis, dysarthria, blurring of vision and even quadriplegia.
6. **List down different type of climate.**
   - Tropical type climate (Sunny)
   - Desert type climate (Very dry)
   - Mediterranean type climate (Mild winter, short wet, warm & dry summer)
   - European type climate (High humidity, result in mist, fog and haze)
   - Monsoon type climate (Typically, winter, summer and rainy seasons)
7. **What is the effect of climate?**
   - It affects indoor & outdoor activities
   - Communication transportation is affected
   - Affects population density and migration of population
   - It affects health and nutritional status of the population
8. **What are all the different methods of continuous chlorination?**
   - Pot diffuser
   - Double Jar diffuser
   - Coconut shell diffuser
9. **Mention the several types of chlorination.**
   - Plain chlorination

- **Pre chlorination** – Raw water chlorination before sedimentation
- **Post chlorination** – After conventional treatment and just before it is supplied to consumer
- **Super chlorination** – Addition of excess chlorine to water as compared to the normal level.
- **De chlorination** – Removal of excess chlorine from water.
- **Break point chlorination** – Addition of chlorine to water in appropriate doses.

10. Define sources of refuse.

- Domestic refuse
- Street refuse
- Industrial refuse
- Constructional refuse
- Hospital refuse
- Stable refuse

11. List down the epidemiological pattern of malaria identified in India.

- Rural malaria
- Urban malaria
- Tribal malaria
- Forest malaria
- Project malaria
- Border malaria

12. Define Malariometry.

It is the measurement of malaria which is done with the help of clinical, parasitology and entomological indexes.

13. What are all the four species of parasites cause malaria in man?

- **Plasmodium vivax** – Cause benign tertian malaria
- **Plasmodium ovale** – Cause ovale tertian malaria
- **Plasmodium malariae** – Cause quartan malaria
- **Plasmodium falciparum** – Cause pernicious malaria

14. Define lepromins.

Lepromins is a mixture of leprosy bacilli and a large quantity of cellular matter derived from lepromatous tissue.

15. List down different type of hepatitis group of viruses.

- Hepatitis A virus (HAV)
- Hepatitis B (HBV)
- Hepatitis C (HCV)
- Hepatitis D (HDV)
- Hepatitis E (HEV)

16. List millennium development goals.

- Eradicate extreme poverty and hunger
- Achieve unusual primary education
- Promote gender equality and empower women (by eliminate gender disparity)
- Reduce child mortality
- Improve maternal health
- Combat HIV/AIDS, malaria and other diseases
- Ensure environmental sustainability
- Develop global partnership for development

17. List down the component of antenatal or prenatal advice.

- **Diet** – Iron rich diet for healthy 12 kg weight gain during pregnancy
- **Personal hygiene** – Include wearing clean cloths, daily bath, clean and tidy hair
- **Rest & sleep** – 8 hours sleep and 2 hours rest
- **Bowels** – avoid constipation by regular intake of green leafy vegetables, fruits extra fluids
- **Exercise** – Light household work
- **Smoking & Alcohol** – Drinking and smoking must be avoided
- **Dental care** – Proper oral hygiene

- **Sexual life** – restricted especially during first and last trimester
- **Drugs** – Certain drugs are discouraged to prevent foetal abnormality
- **Radiation** – Avoid exposure of X-rays during pregnancy
- **Warning signs** – Swelling of feet,, blurring of vision, bleeding it should be reported immediately.
- **Child care** – has to be learnt

18. What are the objectives of postnatal care.

- To prevent complications of postnatal period
- To provide care for rapid restoration of optimum health
- To check adequacy of breast feeding
- To provide family planning services
- To provide basic health education to mother/family

19. List down the complications of the post-natal period.

- **Puerperal sepsis** – Infection of genital tract within 3 weeks after delivery
- **Thrombophlebitis** – Infection of veins of the legs associated with varicose veins

20. List down the recent trends in MCH care.

- Integration of care
- Risk approach
- Manpower changes
- Primary health care

21. List down the elements of (IMCI).

- Assess child for danger sign
- Classify child illness by colour coding triage system
- Identify specific treatment for the child
- Provide practical treatment institutions
- Counsel the mother for any feeding and other problems
- Give follow up care if necessary.

22. Define food hygiene/safety.

WHO defines food hygine as "all conditions and measures that are necessary during the production, processing, storage, distribution and preparation of food to ensure that it is safe, sound, wholesome and fit for human consumption".

23. What are 3 main forms of beriberi.

- Dry form
- Wet beriberi
- Infantile beriberi

24. List down the parameters to evaluate the iron status.

- Haemoglobin concentration
- Serum iron concentration
- Serum ferritin
- Serum transferrin saturation

25. Mention any two breast infections which affect the flow of breast milk.

- Breast abscess
- Mastitis

26. Enumerate reasons why cow's milk is not recommended for a new born.

- It causes allergy
- It may cause GI bleeding and anaemia
- Because it contains too much protein, potassium, sodium, lack of iron and linoleic acid.

27. What are the advantages of women empowerment.

- Better educational status of women
- More employment opportunity
- Economic contribution to the whole family
- Positive change in social attitude
- Increase self esteem
- Increase participation in public meetings and training programmes
- Increasing savings attitude among women. E.g: through SHG, DWACRA group.

28. List down few common chronic illnesses in old age.

- Atherosclerosis
- Hypertension
- Stroke
- Heart attacks
- Cancer
- Diabetes
- Gout
- Rheumatoid arthritis
- Fibrocystic
- Neuritis
- Chronic bronchitis
- Asthma
- Prostate enlargement
- Fibroid uterus

29. Define disaster.

Disaster is "any occurrence, that causes damage, ecological disruption, loss of human life, deterioration of health and health services, on a scale sufficient to warrant an extraordinary response from outside the affected community or area" (WHO, 1995).

30. List down the types of disaster.

Natural Disaster	Man Made
• Hurricanes	Conventional welfare
• Tornados	Non-conventional welfare (e.g. nuclear, chemical)
• Tsunami	Transportation accidents
• Hailstorms	Structural collapse
• Cyclone	Explosions
• Blizzards	Fires
• Drought	Toxin materials
• Foods	Pollution
• Mud slides	Civil
• Earthquakes	Terrorists attacks
• Volcanic eruptions	
• Communicable disease epidemics	

31. List down the formula to calculate weight/height for children.

- The average birth weight of the child in Indian context = 2.7 kg – 2.9 kg
- 3 months to 1 year = $\frac{\text{Age in months} + 9}{2\ (\text{weight in kgs})}$

  or

  Age in months + 11 (weight in lbs)
- 1 – 6 yrs = Age in yrs x 2 + 8 (weight in kg)

  or

  Age in yrs x 5 + 17 = Weight in lbs
- 7 – 12 yrs = $\frac{\text{Age in yrs} \times 7 - 5}{2\ (\text{weight in kgs})}$

  or

  Age in yrs x7 + 5 = weight in lbs
- Formula to calculate Height
  2 – 12 yrs = Age in yrs x 6 + 77

32. What are the ailments common in old age.

- Senile contract
- Nerve deafness
- Osteoporotic changes
- Bronchitis with emphysema
- Changes in mental outlook and many changes.

33. Define community.

Community is a group of individuals who are bound in time and space. They are dependent on each other. They act together for the achievement of common goals. The unit of community is the family.

34. List down the characteristics of health care indicator. Health care indicator should be

- valid
- reliable
- sensitive

- specific
- feasible
- relevant

35. List down the process of community participation.

Motivation

↓ **Creates**

Interest

↓ **Helps in**

Orgainising

↓ **leads to**

Decision Making

↓ **Helps in**

Mobilize

↓

Self Reliance

36. Mention the population covered by rural and tribal PHC.

- **Rural** – For every 30000 population 1 PHC.
- **Tribal** – For every 20000 population 1 PHC.

37. Mention the population covered by rural and urban sub health center

For rural – For every 5000 population one sub center

For tribal – For every 3000 population one sub center

38. What are the therapies comes under manipulation and body based method.

- Chiropractice
- Acupressure
- Acupuncture
- Physiotherapy
- Massage therapy

39. Write any 2 differences between physician and epidemiologist.

Physician	Epidemiologist
Physician will focus on individual/family who are sick.	Epidemiologist will focus upon the whole community.
Physician will focus curative aspect of diseases.	Epidemiologist will focus upon preventing diseases from the community.
Approach of physician is to care of the individual.	Approach of epidemiologist is making comparisons and draw inferences of whole community.
Physician will collect the history of the individual regarding disease condition.	Epidemiologist will collect the history of the affected individuals/ community e.g., his environment and sanitation, etc.

40. What are the occupational diseases caused due to pressure hazard?

- Embolism
- Caisson disease

41. Mention some of the psychological aspect related occupational diseases.

- Neurosis
- Hypertension
- Peptic ulcer
- Dissatisfaction.

42. What are the specialized knowledge and skills needed for occupational nurses?

- First aid and management

- Safety management
- Disaster management
- Toxicology
- Epidemiology
- Environmental sciences and
- Current laws and standards.

43. Mention the classification of chemical hazards.

- Metals (Lead, Arsenic)
- Aromatic hydrocarbons (Benzene, Phenol)
- Aliphatic hydrocarbons (Methyl Alcohol)
- Gases (Co, CH4, etc.)

44. State WHO concept of sexual health.

- H → Happy, healthy mind, healthy body
- E→ Education
- A → Avoid teenage pregnancy
- L → Lactation
- T →Test for pregnancy, RTI, STD
- H → Health screening

45. Write down the acts under MCH services.

- Medical termination of pregnancy act, 1971.
- Child labour Act, 1986.
- Child marriage restraint Act, 1978.
- Hindu adoptions and maintenance act, 1956, for legal adoption upon the child and adoptive parents
- Children act, 1960.
- Juvenile justice act, 1986.

46. Expand RCA and PRAI in sanitary latrines.

RCA – Type of sanitary latrine designed by the Research Cum Action, projects in environmental sanitation of Ministry of Health.

PRAI – Type of sanitary latrine evolved by the Planning Research and Action Institute, Lucknow, Uttar Pradesh.

47. Who is gram sevak?

He is the key person responsible for transforming the economic and social life of the people and he lives with people. His work is to probe people felt need and arouse interest in all round family and village development. He is in charge of 10 villages and attends to 5 or 6 thousand people.

Test Series IX

1. List down the steps in investigation of food poisoning.

- Secure complete list of people involved and collect their history.
- Do the lab investigations. E.g.: Stool and vomit etc.
- Do animal experiments if necessary.
- Take the blood for antibodies.
- Environmental study
- Data analysis

2. List down the components of improving food sanitation.

- Personal hygiene of employees
- Health inspection
- Examine food handlers for infected wounds, diarrhoea, etc.
- Check the food handling technique
- Sanitary improvements
- Health education
- Proper refrigeration
- Surveillance

3. Define the term monitoring in the community.

Monitoring is "the performance and analysis of routine measurements aimed at detecting changes in the environment or health status of population".

4. List down different methods of refuse disposal.

- Hog – feeding (Pigs)
- Stacking or piling up of refuse
- Salvaging (Unhealthy practice)
- Dumping

5. Name sanitary ways of refuse disposal.

- Composting
- Bangalore method
- Sanitary landfill
- Incineration

6. Mention the objectives of housing.

- Shelter
- Safety
- Security
- Privacy

7. What are all the sources of air pollution?

- Industrial sources – Gases, vapours, aerosols
- Automobile sources of lead, oxides of nitrogen, carbon monoxide, ozone etc.
- Agricultural sources e.g . Organo phosporous & organochlorine compounds
- Indoor sources e.g. Sulphur dioxide, tar, ash, etc.
- Natural sources of forest fire, volcanic eruptions, dust storms, sand storms etc.

8. List down the various reasons for anaemia in children.
- Deficient storage due to preterm baby or multi foetal pregnancy
- Inadequate intake
- Diminished absorption
- Increased demand

9. Mention the clinical manifestation of xerophthalmia.
- Night blindness
- Conjuctival xerosis
- Bitot's spots
- Corneal xerosis
- Kerato malacia

10. Mention the kind of equipments used for maintenance of cold chain.
- WIC (Walk in cold room)
- Cold boxes
- Deep freezer big (ILR)
- Various carrier
- SILR small ice lined refrigerator
- Day carrier
- Ice packs

11. List the sanitation of slaughter house.
- It should be away from residential area
- Impervious floor and walls
- Wholesome water supply
- Provision for antemortem & postmortem examination
- Scientific method of collection and disposal of waste
- Rat proof, fry proof, meat storage below 5^0C temperature
- Meat undergo postmortem exam
- Transport of meat in covered containers

12. What are the principles of epidemiology?
- Disease frequency
- Distribution of disease
- Determinants of disease

13. List down the functions of nutritional epidemiology in community health.
- Epidemiological nutritional assessment
- Nutritional and dietary survey
- Nutritional surveillance
- Nutritional and growth monitoring
- Nutritional rehabilitation
- Nutritional indicator and nutritional intervention

14. List down few nutritional status indicators in community.
- Maternal nutrition
- Infant and preschool child nutrition
- School child nutrition

15. List down few milk borne diseases.
- Tuberculosis
- Brucellosis
- Streptococcal infections
- Staphylococcal enterotoxin poisoning
- Q fever
- Cow pox
- Anthrax
- Leptospirosis
- Tick borne encephalitis

16. Define pasteurization of milk.

Pasteurization may be defined as the heating of milk to such temperatures and for such periods of time as are required to destroy any pathogens that may be present while causing minimal changes in the composition, flavour and nutritive value.

17. List down the activities of Applied Nutrition Programme (ANP).
- Supplementary feeding
- Non formal preschool education
- Nutrition education
- Poultry farming
- Beehive keeping
- Providing better seeds, seedlings
- Raising kitchen garden

18. Define food enrichment.

It is the addition of dietary essentials to food to restore the total content of the former. E.g.: Milk with Vit A and D.

19. Define health planning.

It is the orderly process of defining community health problems, identifying unmet needs and surveying the resources to meet those needs, and establishing priority goals that are realistic and feasible and projecting administrative action to accomplish health programmes.

20. List down the elements of planning.

- Objectives
- Policies
- Programmes
- Schedules
- Budget

21. List down the stages of malaria.

- **Cold Stage** – Onset with lassitude, headache, nausea and chills sensation, rise of temperature 39°C – 41°C, skin feels cold and later it becomes hot, rapid pulse. This stage last for ¼-1 hour.
- **Hot Stage** – Skin is hot and dry to touch, full and bounding pulse & rapid respiration. This stage lasts for 2 to 6 hours.
- **Sweating Stage** – Fever comes down with profuse sweating. Skin is cool and moist. The pulse rate becomes slower, feel relief and asleep. This stage lasts for 2-4 hours.

22. Mention the classification of handicapped child.

- **Physically handicapped** – Blind, deaf, mute, hare lip, crippled. E.g.: Polio, burns, accidents etc.
- **Mentally handicapped** – Feeble minded idiots, mental retardation, mental deprivations
- **Psychologically handicapped** – Orphans, maternal deprivation, emotional deprivation, maladjusted child

23. Mention the amount of breast milk secreted for healthy mother per day.

500 – 900 ml of milk/day.

24. Define nipple confusion.

Movement of mouth and tongue are different in breastfeeding and bottle feeding, it will confuse the baby. This is called nipple confusion.

25. Define abortion.

Expulsion of products of conception before viability of foetus (20 to 28 weeks).

26. What is contraceptive method?

Contraceptive methods are defined as a set of methods adopted by women to avoid unwanted pregnancies.

27. List down the characteristics of good contraceptive method.

A good contraceptive method is

- Safe
- Effective
- Acceptable
- Inexpensive
- Reversible
- Simple to administer
- Requires little or no medical supervision

28. Define food safety.

Food safety is the assurance that food will not cause harm to the consumer, when it is prepared or eaten according to its intended use.

29. List down the international health days.

World health day – April 7th
World cancer day – 4th Feb
World heart day – 27th Sep
World sight day – 8th Oct
World DM day – 14th Nov

World Alzheimers day – 21st Sep
World breast feeding week – 1 – 7 Aug
World kidney day – 12 March
World no tobacco day – 31st May
World AIDS day – 1st Dec
World mental health day – 10th Oct
World leprosy day – 31st Jan
Mother's day – 13th May
World TB day – 24th March
World asthma day – 2nd May

30. What is disaster?

D – Destruction
I – Incidents
S – Suffering
A – Administrative financial failures
S – Sentiments
T – Tragedies
E – Eruption of communicable diseases
R – Research programme and implementation

31. List down the principles of disaster management.

The eight basic principles as given by Grab and Eng, 1969 are as follows.

- Prevent the occurrence of the disaster whenever possible.
- Minimize the number of casualties if the disaster cannot be prevented.
- Preventing further casualties after the initial impact of the disaster.
- Rescue the victims.
- Evaluate injured to medical facilities.
- Promote reconstruction of lives.

32. Define eligible couples.

Eligible couple refers to currently married couple, wherein the wife is reproductive age of group (15 – 45 years of age) with one or two living children eligible for adoptions of fertility regulations methods (measure of contraception).

33. Define low birth weight babies.

Low birth weight babies refers to babies whose birth weight is <2500 gm (2.5 kg) .

34. List down the components of health.

- Physical well-being
- Mental well-being
- Social well-being
- Spiritual health

35. Define minor ailments.

Minor ailments are conditions that require either no medical intervention or treatment that can be carried out by the grass roots level health worker.

36. Categorize or classify minor ailments.

- Skin/Mucous membrane ailments
- Aches, pains and discomforts E.g: Body pain, muscle pain, back pain, neck pain, headache etc.
- Respiratory ailments E.g: Nasal congestion, cough colds, flu, choking, etc.
- Alimentary ailments E.g: Ingestion, heart burn, stomach upset, acidity, etc.
- Insects and worms. E.g., Worm infestation, head lice infestation, etc.
- Injuries. E.g: Minor cuts, bruises, burns, minor bleeding.
- Others – Fainting, sleeplessness, nightmares, frequent urination, etc.

37. List down the levels of prevention in community.

- **Primordial prevention** – Health promotion
- **Primary prevention** – Health promotion, specific protection
- **Secondary prevention** – Early detection followed by prompt treatment
- **Tertiary prevention** – Disability limitation, rehabilitation

38. List down few national health programmes in India.

- National antimalaria programme.
- Universal immunization programme
- Reproductive and child health programme
- National tuberculosis control programme.
- National leprosy eradication programme
- National AIDS Control programme
- Integrated Child Development programme
- National diarrhoeal disease control programme
- Vitamin A prophylaxis programme
- National nutritional anemia prophylaxis programme

39. What is principle of magnet therapy?

Every animal, plant has an electromagnetic field that allows other objects to interact as part of one unified energy system.

40. Mention benefits of therapeutic touch.

Wound healing, sleep promotion, enhancement of immune system, decrease anxiety and decrease post-operative pain.

41. What is TLV and TWA?

- TLV – Time threshold limit value
- TWA – Time weighted average

42. What are the types of poisonous gases?

- Simple asphyxiants (N_2, CH_4)
- Chemical asphyxiants (Co, H_2S)
- Irritant (Ammonia, SO_2)
- Systemic poison (CS_2)

43. What are the parasitic and protozoal biological hazard in occupation?

Malaria, hydatid (dog handlers), hook worms, tape worms (agricultural workers)

44. What are the control measures of occupational hazards?

- Medical (Screening, check Up)
- Engineering (Ventilation, substitution, enclosure, isolation, etc)
- Administrative/legal (Legislations)

45. Mention the types of medical statistics.

Health statistics, medical statistics, public health statistics, medicine statistics, vital statistics and demography.

46. What are types of demography?

1. Static demography (Structure of community)
2. Dynamic demography (Functions of community

47. What are the methods of presenting statistical data?

- Tabulation
- Charts and diagrams (pie diagram, pictogram, map diagram, frequency polygon, histogram, etc.)

48. Who are the members of disaster management committee in a school.

- School Principal
- Vice Principal
- Sub divisional magistrate of the area
- DEO (District Educational Officer)
- President of parents teacher association
- Parents (1-2)
- Local medical officer
- Fire officer
- Police
- NSS/NCC/Red cross members
- 4 students

49. State colour coding used in IMNCI.

- **Pink Colour** – Urgent referral
- **Yellow Colour** – Treatment at outpatient health facility and follow up
- **Green Colour** – Home management and follow up

Test Series X

1. **List down attributes of infective agents.**
   - Survivability
   - Resistance
   - Communicability
   - Mutability (genetic change)
   - Infectivity
   - Invasiveness
   - Colonizability
   - Pathogenicity
   - Virulence
   - Immunogenicity
   - Toxigenicity
   - Allergenicity
2. **Define yaws.**
   Yaws is a fast disappearing chronic contagious non venereal, treponema disease of warm and humid regions. Treponema pertenue is the causative organism of yaws.
3. **Define Trachoma.**
   Trachoma is a chronic keratoconjunctivitis affecting conjunctiva producing permanent damage to the sclera. It is essentially a disease of poverty. It is prevalent in those parts of the world where malnutrition is common. Chlamydia trachomatis is the causative agent of trachoma.
4. **Write down the signs and symptoms of chikungunya fever.**
   - Abrupt onset
   - Fever
   - Myalgia
   - Prostration
   - Joint pain
5. **List down the antimalarial drugs.**
   - Chloroquine
   - Proguanil
   - Pyrimethamine
   - Mefloguine
   - Halofantrine
   - Quinine (for multidrug resistant)
   - Primaquine agent tissue schizonts
6. **List down the arrangements you will do for fairs and festivals.**
   - Water supply
   - Conservancy (cleanliness)
   - Food sanitation
   - Accommodation
   - Communication
   - Lighting
   - Medical aid
   - Surveillance
   - Police
7. **Mention the hazards of poor housing.**
   - Respiratory infection
   - Skin infection
   - Arthopod infections

- Accidents
- Increase mortality & morbidity

8. What is nalgonda technique?

The National Environmental Engineering Research Institute, Nagpur has developed a technique for removing fluoride from water by using 2 chemicals (viz. lime and alum) treatment by using sequence of flocculation, sedimentation and filtration of water is called Nalgonda technique.

9. Define food additives.

It is defined as the addition of small quantities of non-nutritious food substances to food and food products to improve the appearance, flavor, texture or storage properties of food.

10. List down the different form of mechanical or artificial ventilation.

- Exhaust ventilation
- Plenum ventilation
- Balanced ventilation
- Air conditioning

11. Define composting.

It is a method of combined disposal of refuse and night soil wherein by natural process, bacterial action results in formation of compost whole is of manorial value to the soil.

12. Define network analysis.

It is a graphic plan of all events and activities to be completed in order to reach an end objective. It brings greater discipline in planning.

13. List down the general functions of DGHS (Director General of Health Services).

- Survey
- Planning & coordination
- Programming
- Appraisal of health matters

14. List down the steps of food sanitation.

- Meat inspection
- Personal hygiene
- Screening of food handlers
- Proper food handling technique
- Health education
- Sanitation improvement
- Mention the organism for amoebiasis.

Amoebiasis is a protozoal infection and it is caused by entamoeba histolytica

15. List down the community control measures of amoebiasis.

- Sanitation – Safe disposal of excreta
- Chlorinated pure water supply
- Maintaining food hygiene including washing vegetables
- Screening of food handlers
- Health education
- Early diagnosis
- Early treatment

16. Specify the mode of transmission of amoebiasis.

- **Faecal** – Oral Route – By contaminated water or food
- **Sexual transmission** – Oral – rectal by sexual transmission
- **Vectors** – Flies, cockroaches & rodents capable of carrying cyst

17. List down the prevention and control of hookworm infection.

- Sanitary disposal of faeces
- Chemotherapy
- Treatment of anaemia
- Health education

18. List down mode of transmission of rabies.

- Animal bites
- Licks
- Aerosols
- Person to person

19. Write the local treatment for rabies.

- Isolate the infected person

- Cleaning the wound with soap and water
- Chemical treatment of wound E.g.: Iodine/Povidine
- Suturing the wound
- Antirabies serum
- Antibiotics and antitetanus measure
- Observe the animal for 10 days

20. List down the indications for antirabies treatment.

It should be started immediately.

- If the animal shows signs of rabies or it dies within 10 days of observation.
- If the biting animal cannot be identified.
- Unprovoked bites
- Laboratory tests e.g:, blood of biting animal are tested for rabies
- All bites by wild animals.

21. What is chikungunya fever, what are all the symptoms?

It is dengue like disease caused by a group A virus, the chikungunya virus is transmitted by aedes, culex and mansonia mosquitoes with the clinical symptoms of high fever, and severe articular pains in the limbs and spinal column.

22. Mention the two main organization is responsible for BFH Initiative.

- WHO
- UNICEF

23. List down the contra indications of breast feeding.

- Illegal drug use
- Active untreated tuberculosis
- HIV positive mother
- hemotherapy
- Herpetic lesions on the breast

24. What is the epidemiology of disaster?

Epidemiology is the study of pattern of disease occurrence in human populations and the factors that influence these patterns. It may be studied and analyzed using the epidemiological framework of agent, host and environment in an attempt to predict, prevent or control the outcomes of disaster, both natural and man-made.

25. List down the phases of disaster.

- **Pre Impact Phase** – Initial prior to the actual occurrence of disaster
- **Impact Phase** – Disaster actually happened
- **Post Impact Phase** – (4 stages)
- Denial
- Strong emotional response
- Acceptance
- Recover

26. List down three major management of LBW babies.

- Prevention of hypothermia
- Promotion of exclusive breast feeding
- Prevention of infections

27. What is secondary post partum haemorrhage?

It occurs after 24 hrs or within 42 days of the delivery.

28. List down the causes of secondary postpartum haemorrhage.

- Retained bits of placenta
- Infection
- Inversion of uterus
- Placental polyp
- Mention ideal postnatal visit.

Advice the mother as follows

- Atleast two postnatal visits are must
- **First visit** – within 10 days of delivery
- **Second visit** – 6 weeks of delivery

29. List down the aims of the 1st postnatal visit.

Aims of first visit

- Obtain history on
- Delivery
- Bowel & bladder function
- Sleep, lactation etc.
- For general examination for fever, anaemia, BP, uterus, breast etc.
- To examine the normal size of uterus and its involution etc.

30. List down the main aim of second post-natal visit.
- Study the involution of uterus
- Assess Hb levels
- Screen for fitness for contraception

31. List down the few older theories or concepts of disease condition.
- Supernatural theory
- Tridosha theory of disease causation
- The Greek Humoral theory
- Germ theory of disease causation
- The body machine and the mind theory

32. List down the factors influencing community health.
- Socio-cultural factors
- Political factors
- Economic system
- Religious system
- Education system
- Environmental system
- Health care system

33. List down the goal of community health nursing.
- Health promotion
- Health maintenance
- Disease prevention
- Treatment and restoration of health
- Rehabilitation

34. List down the 10 subsystem in community.
- Health
- Family
- Economic
- Education
- Welfare
- Political
- Legal
- Religion
- Recreation
- Communication

35. Mention the Kurt Lewins stages of change.
- Unfreezing stage
- Freezing stage (Here the community health nurse acts as a change agent)
- Refreezing

36. List down nutritional health problems in India.

Low birth weight, protein energy malnutrition, xerophthalmia, nutritional anaemia, iron deficiency disorders, endemic fluorosis, lathyrism.

37. Mention the types of yoga.

Karma yoga
Bhakti yoga
Jnana yoga and
Raja yoga

38. State the advantages and disadvantages of herbal therapy.

Advantages:
- Fewer side effects
- Amendable to self care
- Lower cost

Disadvantages:
- Long time to get the onset of action
- Possible drug herb interaction
- Inconsistent manufacturing practices

39. What are the benefits under ESI Act?
- Medical Benefit
- Sickness Benefit
- Maternity Benefit
- Dependent's Benefit

40. What are the provisions of factories act, 1946?

- Employment provision
- Welfare provision
- Safety provision
- Sanitary provision

41. Who is the father of occupational health?

Bernardino Ramazzini (1633-1714)

42. Define occupational hazard.

Source/situation with a potential for harm in terms of injury or ill health, damage to property, damage to the work place environment or a combination of these.

43. Mention the collection of vital statistics in various hierarchy levels.

Bureau of Health Statistics (State)

↓

Director General of Health Services (National)

↓

WHO regional office (South East Asia)

↓

WHO head office (Geneva)

↓

United Nations (International Level)

44. Mention the objectives of 20 point programme.

- Eradication of poverty
- Raising productivity
- Reducing inequalities
- Removing social & economic disparities
- Improving the quality of life

45. Define sex ratio.

It is defined as "the number of females per 1000 males". It is the basic demographic characteristics of population.

46. Define abortion ratio.

This is calculated by dividing the number of abortions performed during a particular time period by the number of live births over the same period.

47. Define dependency ratio.

The proportion of persons above 65 yrs of age and children below 15 yrs of age are considered to be dependent on the economically productive age group (15-64 years).

48. What do you mean by emerging and re-emerging diseases with examples?

Emerging diseases refers to newly appearing infectious diseases or diseases that are spreading to new geographical areas such as cholera, yellow fever, etc.

Reemerging diseases refers to the diseases which were previously easily controlled by chemotherapy and antibiotics, but they have developed antimicrobial resistance are often appearing in epidemic form e.g., malaria, neisseria gonorrhoea/chikengunya.

COMMUNICATION AND EDUCATION TECHNOLOGY

INTRODUCTION

Communication and educational technology is the combination of the concepts of both communication and the application of educational ideas. An excellent educational technology, if imparted to the learner without proper communication, is considered as mere waste.

Human relation and interpersonal relationship

The Nurse is an important health team member who has to work in harmony for the care of the patient. This cooperation is dependent upon the interpersonal relationship that is maintained among the health care team members.

Guidance and Counselling

Everyone in this world encounters problems one or the other day. These problems can be solved by the individual. Sometimes a person with problems may seeks professionals help to solve these problems. The students of nursing education are adolescents most of the times. One wrong move during this period may, lands the student in a many critical situations. Therefore it is important for guidance and Counselling in order to make the best choices for life and career.

Teaching learning process

Learning is essential to replenish knowledge. Students have to play a dominant role in the learning process, whereas the role of the teacher is limited to a facilitator or stage setter. Education is a natural, harmonious and progressive development of man's innate powers (Pestalozzi). Philosophy of nursing education is a perfect combination of philosophy of nursing and education. Philosophy will decide the nature of student selection process, objectives of educational programs, curriculum development, type of experiences provided, staff selection and evaluation system.

Methods of teaching

Teaching nursing also involves effective application of different teaching learning methods, some of which are specially designed to impart knowledge and clinical skills essential for a successful nursing career. There are various methods of teaching that are employed in nursing to teach theory and clinical skills.

A.V aids

Technology explosion has yielded a several new machines, materials and media, which have a great potential for the use in the educational process. A judicious use of these together with teaching learning led to the development of new field called educational technology. Educational technology is a system in education in which machines, materials, media and men work together to achieve educational objectives.

Evaluation

Education is considered necessary to bring about changes in the behaviour of an individual. So it is important to evaluate the educational process periodically. Based on the frequency ofn conducting evaluation, it can be formative or summative. There are various tools that are used to assess the educational objectives.

Health education

Information, education and communication includes various approaches that enable individuals and group such as family, community to play active role in maintaining health. Health behavior is dependent on various factors like family, literacy, religion, beliefs, customs etc.

References

1. Sankaranarayanan S, Sindhu B.(2012.) **Learning and Teaching Nursing**. 4th ed. Jaypee.
2. Neeraja KP. (2003). **Textbook of Nursing Educaion**. 1st ed. Jaypee.
3. Sheeba T, Prasanna ML. (2011). **Communication and Educational Technology**. 2nd ed. Frontline.

Test Series I

1. **Classify attitude.**
   Facilitating attitude
   Inhibiting attitude
2. **What is the process of human interaction through communication?**
   - Verbal and non-verbal
   - Written and unwritten
   - Planned and unplanned
3. **List down few features that help the nurses in communication skill.**
   - Generate link between nurse and client
   - Provide the nurse with professional satisfaction
   - Communication provide means of coordination
   - Communication serves as a channel for fostering the smooth operation
4. **Define two-way communication.**
   A good communication system must contain a feedback mechanism. The sender should try to know the reaction of the receiver. This will enable the management to know whether or not message is received.
5. **What is 'The Best Model'?**
   It is the model for employing communication in real settings:
   - Begin with non-verbal cue
   - Establish information gathering with informal talk.
   - Support with emotional chance
   - Terminate.
6. **Enlist communication system being used in hospitals.**
   - Periodic talk between employer and employee.
   - Message gathering
   - Employee Counselling
   - Murals
   - Bulletin board
7. **Present the acronym 'SOLER'.**
   - S-Sit squarely facing the patient
   - O-Observe an open posture
   - L-Lean forward toward the patient
   - E-Establish eye contact
   - R-Relax whether sitting or standing during interaction
8. **List down the qualities of good listener.**
   - Face the person who talks
   - Maintain good eye contact
9. **What are the basic communication skills?**
   Human relation skills
   Listening skills
   Active listening
   Writing and reading skill

Drawing attention skill

10. Define feedback.

It is the message that the receiver return to the sender. It helps the sender to recognize whether the meaning of his message has been received as intended.

11. Define communication.

Communication is a process by which two or more people exchange ideas, facts, feelings or impressions in ways that each gains a common understanding of meaning intend and use of a message –Paul Leo gens.

12. What are the influences of the communication by a communicator?

- The words we have at our command
- The way we put them together it affect, how we think about
- Whether we are thinking at all

13. Define attitude.

It is the tendency or predisposing act in a particular direction to a thing, person or an event.

14. What are the factors influence the effectiveness of the communication?

- Communication skills
- Knowledge
- Attitudes
- Position with in the socio cultural system of the country in which the person lives.

15. List barriers in effective communication.

- Personal
- Physical implements
- Mechanical factors
- Educational difference
- Rumours
- Organizational barriers
- Large institution

16. Compare one way and two way communication.

One way	Two way
Is considerably faster than two way	More accurate
Appears neat and efficient	More people use this method
Accuracy less	Relatively noisy and disorderly with people interrupting the sender and one another
Sender is more psychologically comfortable	Much more a trial and error method

17. What is 'psychic communication?

Extra sensory perception occurs about something which will occur in future for the person

18. List the components of a message.

The components of the message are:

- Message code
- Message content
- Message treatment

19. Enlist the principles of communication.

- Communication should be appropriate to situation
- Communication should have objectives and purpose
- Communication should promote achievement of purpose

20. What is serial communication?

Person to person the message will be passed like a chain. Senders pass the message to one person, then that receiver passes information to other and so on.

21. Specify the objectives of a communication.

- Awareness of information
- Action information
- Continuing information

- Updating information

22. List the purpose of communication.

- To transfer information between all classes of employees, to have a common understanding among them.
- To interpret and adopt policies in the organization.

23. What is the importance of communication?

- It reduces the interpersonal tensions and improves the interpersonal relationship.
- Poor communication results in poor patient care and poor interpersonal relationships.

24. Describe communication process.

Elements of communication:

- Sender
- Message
- Channel
- Receiver
- Feedback

25. Enlist the forms of communication.

- Verbal communication
- Non-verbal communication

26. Mention the purposes of communication in Nursing.

- To Transfer information between all classes of employees to have a common understanding among them.
- To improve employee-employer relationship.

27. Enlist types of non-verbal communication.

a) Physical appearance
b) Posture and gait
c) Facial expression
d) Eye contact
e) Body movements
f) Touch
g) Tone of voice

28. What are the results of effective communication nursing?

The needs of communication are

It generates trust between the nurse and clients

Provides the trust between nurses with professional satisfaction.

It is a means for bringing about change.

It is a foundation of relationship between the nurse and other member of the health team.

29. Differentiate formal and informal communication.

Formal communication	Informal communication
Formal communication is officially organized channel of communication and it is delayed communication	The informal communication channels may be more active if the normal channels do not cater the information needs.
It is according to the prescribed or fixed norms or rules or customs	It may be fact but more in nature of rumor

30. List down disadvantages of oral communication:

- The spoken words may be misunderstood.
- The facial expression and tone of voice of the communicator may mislead the receiver
- Not suitable for lengthy communication. It requires the art of effective speaking.

31. List down 4 advantages of oral communication.

- It is face to face system and hence doubts can be clarified.
- There is an opportunity to ask ques-

tions, exchange ideas and clarify meanings.

- It can develop a friendly and cooperative spirit.
- It is easy and quick.

32. List advantages of written communication.

- It is permanent record for future references
- It is less likely to be misunderstood.
- It will have adequate coverage and accuracy. It is an authoritative communication

33. List disadvantages of written communication.

- It requires skill education for understanding
- It is one-way communication and hence not effective.

34. List essentials of good communication.

- Avoid technical words and abbreviation that are not in use.
- Pay attention to the non verbal message accompanying the verbal messages.
- The sender and receiver use the same language and express ideas in simple words.
- There should be clarity in expressing ideas.

35. List the basic skills of communication.

- Human relation skills
- Active listening skills
- Writing and reading skills
- Drawing skills

36. List the communication systems in hospital.

- Periodic talks between employee and employer.
- Staff conferences.
- Standing orders, protocols
- Hospital magazine
- Annual reports.

37. How to overcome communication barriers.

- Clarify the idea
- Completeness of the message
- Understand the receiver
- Use appropriate channels
- Consistency in communication

38. What are the commandments of good communication?

- Seek to clarify your ideas before communicating
- Examine the true purpose of easy communication before communicating.

39. What are the essentials of sound communication?

- Clarity
- Adequacy
- Right timing
- Integrity
- Participation
- strategic use of grapevine

40. List down the types of reasoning.

- Inductive reasoning is the drawing of a general conclusion from a consideration of particular cases.
- Deductive reasoning is drawing of a conclusion from general principles to specific.

41. List the steps in problem solving.

- Recognizing the problem
- Defining the problem
- Formulating possible and relevant answer to the problem.
- Testing the selected answer
- Formulating conclusions.

42. List the ways of thinking.

- Reasoning
- Problem-solving

- Critical thinking
- Creative thinking

43. What are the elements of the learning process?

- Goal
- Stimulus
- Perception
- Response
- Consequence
- Integration

44. What are all the conceptual approaches in learning?

- Clinical philosophical
- Field theory
- Association theory
- Structure theory

45. List any four types of communication.

- One-way communication
- Two-way communication
- Verbal communication
- Mechanical communication

46. Write two strategies of a communication?

The words we have at our command
Whether we are thinking at all

47. List two physical barriers in effective communication?

- Language
- Cultural factors

48. Enlist the components of communication.

- Sender (Source)
- Message
- Channel
- Receiver

49. Specify the two objectives of communication.

- Awareness of information
- Action information

Test Series II

1. **Define therapeutic nurse-patient relationship.**
   Nurse-client relationship is a helping relationship that is therapeutic in nature and is established to meet the needs of clients and is based on trust and respect.
2. **List down the types of relationships.**
   - Social relationship
   - Intimate relationship
   - Therapeutic relationship
3. **Differentiate social and therapeutic relationship.**
   Social relationship:
   It is the most common kind of relationship both individual are usually involved in the relationship and are concerned with meeting their own needs.
   Therapeutic relationship:
   The nurse and client work together to meet the goal of assisting the client to regain the their resource to meet the life challenges and facilitate the growth.
4. **What are the phases of therapeutic relationship?**
   - Pre-interaction phase
   - Orientation phase
   - Working phase
   - Termination phase
5. **List the principles of interpersonal relationship.**
   - Learn everyone's name and never address anyone by any nick name
   - Respect everyone's individually. Each member of a team is as important as other.
   - Do not impose over anything on anybody
   - Keep emotions under control
6. **Write any four role of nurse in therapeutic communication.**
   - Helping the client to identify what is troubling the client.
   - Encourage to discuss about the changes needed to make in the client
   - Assist the client to select an alternative
   - Provide positive feedback for the clients attempt to create changes.
7. **Enlist the conditions used in therapeutic relationship.**
   i. Rapport
   ii. Trust
   iii. Respect
   iv. Genuineness
   v. Empathy
   vi. Power
   vii. Intimacy

8. Specify any four elements of professional communication.

- Being on time
- Courtesy
- Use of names
- Privacy & confidentiality

9. List down any 4 purpose of communication.

- It should be expressed in terms of human behavior
- It should be specific
- It should be consistent
- It is not logically contraindicated

10. List down the goals of therapeutic relationship.

- Facilitates communication of distressing thoughts and feelings
- To assist client's in problem solving to help daily living
- Help client examine self detecting behavior and test alternatives
- Promote self-care and independence

11. List down any 4 therapeutic communication techniques.

- Using silence
- Using touch
- Giving information
- Reflecting

12. Define communication.

Communication is a process by which two or more people exchange ideas, facts, feelings or impressions in ways that each gains a common understanding of meaning, intent and use of message- Paul Leo gens.

13. List the ways of communication.

- Oral or written
- Sign/ signal or symbol
- Action
- Object

14. List the objectives of communication.

- Awareness of information
- Action information
- Continuing information
- Updating information

15. Specify the components of communication.

- Source
- Message
- Channel
- Receiver

16. List down any four types of communication.

- One way communication
- Interpersonal communication
- Physiological communication
- Verbal communication

17. Enlist the barriers of effective communication.

- Mechanical factors
- Educational difference
- Rumors
- Personal barriers
  - Language
  - Age and sex

18. List any 4 principles of communication.

- Communication should share information
- Communication should be appropriate to situation
- Communication should have objectives and purpose
- Communication should promote total achievement of purpose

19. Specify any 4 qualities of a good communicator.

- He knows how to organize and treat his message
- He is interested in audience and its welfare
- He prepares and plan for communication
- He plan and evaluate the results

20. List down components of johari window model.
- Arena
- Blind spot
- Facade
- Unknown

21. How to improve or increase the size of the arena?
- Arena relating to others by the behavioral processes, you choose to use in your relationships.
- Reducing the facade

22. What are all the two key ideas behind the johari window model?
- That individual can build trust between themselves by disclosing information about themselves.
- That they can learn about themselves and come to terms with personal issues with the help of feedback from others.

23. Define arena.

In Johari window model, the arena is the portion of the total interpersonal space devoted to mutual understanding and shared information. This is known by the self-known by other facet of the relationship is thought to control interpersonal productivity.

24. Define facade.

Facade in Johari window represents the "hidden quadrants" things that I know about myself that you do not know.

25. Define blind spot in johari window model.

The blind quadrant represents things that you know about me, but I am unaware of so.

26. What are all the skills of communication?
- Encoding skills
- Speaking and writing
- Decoding skills-listening and reading
- Intellectual skills-perceiving, memorizing.

27. List the factors influencing the skills of a communicator.
- The words we have at our command
- The way we put them together
- Whether we are thinking at all

28. What are all the three components of message?
- Message code
- Message content
- Message treatment

Test Series III

1. **What the factors affecting self concept.**
   - Early bonding experiences
   - Personality characteristics
   - Culture
   - Environment
   - Socio economic status
   - Interpersonal and personal roles.
2. **What are the components of self concept?**
   - Self concept
   - Extend self
   - Desired self
   - Presenting self
3. **What are the stages of psychosocial development?**
   - Trust Vs mistrust
   - Autonomy Vs doubt and shame
   - Initiative Vs guilt
   - Industry Vs inferiority
   - Identity Vs identity confusion
   - Intimacy Vs isolation
   - Generativity Vs stagnation
   - Integrity Vs despair.
4. **Define group.**
   Group is defined as a unit of analysis in group dynamics is of almost importance. It is a social unit which has been variously defined.
5. **What are the characteristics of group?**
   - Membership in group
   - Emergent in leadership
   - Formal hierarchy
   - Group has some activity or task to perform
   - Interaction
   - Group norm
6. **List down any two principles of group dynamics.**
   The more attractive a group to its member, the greater the influence it would exercise on its members.
   The greater the prestige on a group member in the eyes of other member, the greater the influence he will exercise on them.
7. **What are all the nature of team work?**
   - A team group
   - A leader
   - A common goal
   - Regular interaction
   - Each member's contributing responsibility
   - Coordination
   - Team spirit
8. **List down the tools and issues that support team.**
   - In group and out group
   - Power and control
   - Appreciation for individual skills

- Group agreement

9. What are the concepts of self concept development?

- Symbolic interactions
- Developmental task
- Self concept stability
- Locus of control.

10. Define primary group.

Primary group is characterized by intimate face to face association and coordination.

11. What is the definition of self concept?

Self concept is the composite of beliefs and feelings that one holds about oneself at a given time, formed from perception particularly of others reactions or behavior. Theories of self and growth and development.

- Erickson's psychosocial development
- Freud theory
- Sullivan theory
- Paget theory
- Kohlberg theory

12. List down the criteria for a group.

- Formal and social structure
- Face to face interaction
- Two or more persons
- Common fate
- Common goals
- Interdependence
- Self definition as a group members
- Recognition by others.

13. List the types of groups.

- Formal group
- Informal group

According to purpose:

- Vocational groups
- Instructional groups
- Government groups
- Religious groups
- Functional groups
- Recreational groups
- Social groups

14. List the stages of group development.

- Forming
- Storming
- Norming
- Performing
- Adjourning

15. Define of team work.

A team as a group of people with a high degree of interdependence geared toward the achievement of a goal or task.

16. List 4 indications of bad team work.

- Frustration
- Grumbling and retaliation
- Unhealthy competition
- Dishonesty and lack of openness

17. Specify the key concept of team?

- Communication
- Mission
- Willingness to cooperate
- Commitment.

18. What is stages of psychosexual development?

Infancy (birth to 1year) – Oral
Toddler (1- 3year) – Anal
Preschool (6-12year) – Phallic
Schooler (6-12 year) – Latency
Adolescent (12-19year)-Genital

19. Define secondary group.

Secondary groups are those where the interrelationship are more general and remote. The membership to such group is generally voluntary and easily withdrawable.

20. What is physical self- image?

It is usually formed first and is related to the child's physical appearance, its attractiveness and its self appropriateness and importance of the different parts of the body to behavior and to the percentage they give the child in the eyes of others.

21. What is self esteem?

Self esteem refers to the degree of regard or respect that individuals have for them and is a measure of worth that they place on their abilities and judgment. Self esteem is closely related to the other components of the self concept. Just as with image and personal identity the development of self esteem is largely influenced by the eruptions of how one is viewed by significant others.

22. What is personal body image?

An individual body image is a personal appraisal of his or her physical being and includes physical attributes, functioning, serenity, wellness-illness state and appearance. It is an integration of collections of visual, auditory, tactile and proprioceptive information that combines with effective and cognitive process to form image of one's physical self.

23. What is group?

According to humans, group is a number of persons who communicate with one another, often over a span of time and who are few enough so that each person is able to communicate with all the others not at second hand, though others not at second hand through other people but face to face.

24. Mention the types of formal group.

- Command group
- Task group
- Permanent formal groups
- Temporary or momentary groups.

25. What are concept and theories of infancy?

Concept	Infancy(1-12months)
Challenge	Trust Vs mistrust
Significant	Funnily cargneces
Necessary accomplishment	Development
Virtues	Hope
Ways to help the child succeed	Establish routine, satisfy basic needs

26. What are the theories of psychological development in toddlerhood?

Concept	Toddlerhood (1-3yr)
Challenge	Autonomy Vs shame and doubt
Significant	Family
Development	Learn appropriate behavior
Necessary	Learn right from wrong.
Accomplishment Virtues	Self control, will power
Ways to help the child succeed	Set limits let child make simple choices Encourage curiosity give gentle guidance

27. What are all the theories of psychological development in preschool children?

Concept	Preschool (3-6yr)
Challenge	Imitative Vs guilt
Significant	Family
Necessary accomplishment	Learn rules and regula tions establish independence.
Virtues	Direction, purpose.
Way to help the child succeed	Consistent discipline, explain things, praise.

28. What are stages of Piaget and Kohl berg?

Infant (birth to 1year)

Infant (continued)

Early childhood (continued)
Late childhood (6-9 years)
Early childhood (continued)
Late childhood (6-9 years)
Early childhood (12-15years)
Kohl berg stages of moral development
Pre conventional (Birth to 7years)
Reconvention
Conventional (7-12years)
Post conventional (12years and older)

29. What are all the theories of development in school age?

Concept	School Age (6-12 Years)
Challenge	Industry Vs inferiority
Significant	School and neighborhood
Necessary accomplishment	Learn to get along with others learn school subjects
Virtues	Self esteem, competence
Way to help the child succeed	Manage siblingrivalry give responsibility recognize accomplishment away from home.

30. What is intimacy versus isolation?

The young adult makes commitment to another, moves from the relative security of self identify to the relative in security involved in establishing intimacy with another. Those with a poor sense of self tend to have less committed relationships and are more likely to suffer emotional isolation, loneliness and depression. The psychological strength during young adult is love.

31. What are the two types of group?

Primary group: It is characterized by face to face association and coordination.

Non-primary or secondary groups: Are those where the inter relationships are more general and remote. The membership to such group is generally voluntary and easily withdrawable.

32. What are the three different kinds of groups which are found in organization?

i. Horizontal groups
ii. Vertical groups
iii. Mixed or random groups

33. What are the characteristics of effective team?

- The working atmosphere is informal comfortable, and relaxed
- There are no obvious people who are involved and interested.
- These is lot of discussion in which virtually everyone participates to the task of the group. If the discussion gets off the subjects someone will bring it back on track shortly.

34. What are the attributes of effective and ineffective team?

Attribute	effective team	Ineffective team
Working Environment	Informal, comfortable relaxed	Ineffective, bored, Fuse and stiff
Discussions	Focused, should by almost everyone	Frequently, unfocused, documented by a few.

35. What are the group agreements?

a) Trust
b) Team spirit
c) Leadership skills

d) Nurse manger's role

36. What are advantages of patient care delivery system?

Each person became very efficient at specific tasks and a great amount of work can be done in short time.

Unskilled workers can be trained to perform one or two specific tasks very well.

By decreasing the number of registered nurses, the hospital has fewer personnel cost.

37. What are the disadvantages of the patient care delivery system?

The patient becomes confused with so many different care provides per shift.

Poor communication almost has no improvement or problems of patient state as one care provides seen patient care from beginning to the end.

Poor leadership skills of the team leader.

38. What are the indications for bad teamwork?

I. Frustrations
II. Grumbling and retaliation
III. Unhealthy competition
IV. Miserable facial expression of employees
V. Dishonesty and lack of openness

Test Series IV

1. **What is the meaning of the word 'Guide'?**
   - To indicate
   - To point out
   - To show the way
   - To lead
   - To direct
   - To seek
2. **Define guidance.**
   Guidance is a process of dynamic interpersonal relationship designed to influence the attitudes and subsequent behavior of a person –Good.
   Guidance is a process through which an individual is able to solve their problems and aspirations – JM Brewer.
3. **List the elements of guidance.**
   It focuses our attention on the individual and not the problem.
   Guidance leads to the discovery of abilities of an individual.
   Guidance is based upon the assets and limitations of an individual.
4. **Which elements of guidance focuses to improve student's capacity?**
   Educational-Social
   Moral-Emotional
   Vocational-Avocational
   Health -Leisure activity.
5. **List the characteristics of guidance.**
   It is a continuous process.
   Choice and problem points are the distinctive concerns of guidance.
   It is both generalized and specialized.
6. **Explain the principles of guidance.**
   Guidance services which are aimed at bringing about desirable adjustment in any particular area of experience must be taken into account the all round development of the individual.
   Guidance touches every phase of an individual life pattern.
7. **List the need for guidance.**
   - Complex nature of society
   - Individual differences
   - Welfare, safety of an individual
   - Changed industrial and educational pattern of the country.
   - Changed economic patterns of the country.
   - Conservation of the human energy.
8. **What are all the process of complex nature of society?**
   - Consumption
   - Production
   - Distribution
   - Exchange.

9. What is the necessary of guidance for good citizenship?
- Study habits and skills
- Career choice/vocational choice
- Knowledge of aptitudes and abilities
- Sex education
- Family relationship
- Mental hygiene

10. List down the areas of guidance.
- Curricular and co-curricular choice.
- Acquire basic study skills for optimum achievements.
- Spend leisure properly.
- Adjust to the peers and parents, teachers, administrators.

11. When recreational guidance is needed?
Recreational guidance is needed when an individual wants to choose the type of recreation and wants to assess the resources required and their competency to perform. Recreational guidance will also help them to choose based on the various needs for recreation namely physical, emotional, intellectual, social, environmental and spiritual dimensions.

12. List the purpose of group guidance.
- To permit each individual in the group to solve his problem.
- To make necessary adjustment.
- To improve student's attitude and behavior.
- To give training for the students in different aspects of leadership.

13. What is the need for group guidance in education?
- Counsellor may save time by group approach.
- Able to pay more attention to more difficult and complex aspects of the situation faced by an individual student.
- Gives opportunity to the students to express their unexpressed feelings.
- It helps the participants to achieve better balanced judgments by few exchange of opinions, realistic analysis of attitudes.

14. List principles of group guidance.
It should be a supplement to counselling not a substitute for it. It encourages certain member of the group to seek individual Counselling help. Group should be homogeneous in various aspects. Appropriate project to the students should be introduced.

15. List the techniques of group guidance.
- Talk
- Career conferences
- Audio-visual aids
- Visits
- Group activities
- Occupational information through school subjects
- Informal discussion
- Group reports
- Lectures
- Discussion
- Question bank
- Case conferences.

16. List the types of talks in group guidance.
- General orientation talks
- Educational orientation talks
- Vocational orientation talks
- Personal-social adjustment orientation talk

17. What is the purpose for case conference in group guidance?
It supplements the information given to a group to explain the vocation in which they work. Providing information about the advantages and disadvantages of differ-

ent occupations and courses, qualifications necessary for entry in to them and the range of opportunities available.,

18. List the kinds of groups for group guidance.

- Regular subject groups
- Typical group
- Career or educational groups
- Groups with common interest

19. Mention any four advantages of group guidance?

- Economical and efficient
- Helps in having more contacts with students
- Opportunity to discuss common problem
- Helps to improve student's attitudes and behaviour.

20. What is the use of question box in group guidance?

It gives the pupil an opportunity to propose a question and is used as vocation guidance to the student

21. What are the major guidance and counselling areas?

- Education
- pre-admission guidance needs
- post-admission guidance needs
- Vocation
- occupation
- Social guidance
- Guidance related to health
- Moral guidance
- Personal guidance
- Marital guidance

22. What are types of guidance?

- Educational guidance
- Vocational guidance
- Guidance in social and civic activities
- Guidance in health and physical activities
- Guidance in worthy use of leisure time
- Guidance in character building.

23. Define educational guidance.

It is a process concerned with bringing about between the individual pupil with his distinctive characteristics for one hand, and differing of opportunities and requirement in the other, a favourable setting for the individual's development of education.

24. List some of the objectives of educational guidance.

- Physical, emotional and social, mental development of the individual
- Provision of health
- Command of fundamental process.
- Worthy home membership.

25. Mention the problems of educational guidance.

To help the individual to make desirable progress in his educational career.

26. Define personal guidance.

The guidance offered to the individual to solve his emotional, social, ethical and moral as well as the health problems.

27. Define vocational guidance.

It is the process of assisting the individual to choose an occupation, prepare for it enter upon and progress in it.

28. What is the aims of vocational guidance?

Acquire the knowledge of characteristics, functions, duties, responsibilities, rewards of the group of occupation.

Discover his own potentials, abilities and skills

To think critically about various types of occupations.

Provides information about the problem

29. What is the nature and purpose of personal guidance?

- It deals with all problems of life
- It is concerned with social and civic activities
- It is also concerned with the worthy use of leisure time, physical activities.
- It has major concern for individual and social problems.

30. What are the stages of personal guidance?

- Pre-primary stage
- Elementary stage
- Junior high school stage
- High school stage
- College and university stage

31. Define counselling.

Counselling is a method that help the client use a problem solving process to recognize and manage stress and that facilitates inter personal relationship among client, family and health care team.

32. What are the elements in counselling process?

Counselling involves two individuals

Counsellor–A professionally trained person who can assist or help the counseled.

Counselee – A person who seeks help or need assistance.

33. What are the principles followed in counselling technique?

- Acceptance
- Re-assurance
- Clarification
- Resource
- Interpretation
- Advice
- Rejection
- Lead

34. What are the phases of counselling?

Phase 1: Establishing relationship

Phase 2: Assessment

Phase 3: Setting goals

Phase 4: Intervention

Phase 5: Termination and follow up

35. What are the steps in counselling?

- Analysis
- Synthesis
- Diagnosis
- Prognosis
- Counselling
- Follow up

36. What are characters of counsellor?

- Friendly nature
- Gets along with other
- Sympathetic understanding
- Fairness
- Attentive listener
- Maintain external stability
- Positive interest
- Respects the facts

37. What are the characteristics of counselling?

- It is a purposeful learning experience for the counselee
- It is a purpose oriented and private interview between the counsellor and counselee.
- Based on mutual confidence, satisfactory relationship will be established.
- Counselling process is structured around the felt needs of the counselee.

38. What are the needs of counselling?

- To encourage and develop special abilities and right attitudes.
- To inspire successful end towards attainment.
- To assist the students in planning for educational and vocational choices.
- To help the student to grow, explore and maintain their overall personality.
- To help the student in need of special help.

39. List the principles of counselling.

- Tailor made to the requirement of an individual problem.
- Emphasize thinking with the individual
- Avoid dictating attitude
- Maintain relationship of trust and confidence with the client.
- Client's need is to be put first

40. What are the types of counselling?

- Directive Counselling
- Non directive Counselling
- Short term Counselling
- Long term Counselling
- Elective Counselling
- Clinical Counselling
- Psychological Counselling

41. What is the concepts of counselling?

- Counselling is a relationship between two persons one of them at assist the other in organizing himself to attain a form of happiness, adjustment to a life situation.
- To develop a set of goals or behavior of an individual.
- Helps the individual to discuss the problems and acquire social skills, courage etc.
- The relationship between two personal who require help from the skilled person to resolve his problems.

42. What are the process of effective counselling?

- Counselling is not filling the information, though information may be present.
- Counselling is not filing an advice.
- Counselling is not the selection and assignment of individual to job.
- Counselling is not interviewing, though interviewing is involved.

43. What are the levels of Counselling?

Informal counselling
Professional
Non specialist counselling by professionals.

44. Enumerate the aspects of Counselling?

- Collection of information.
- Careful analysis of the available facts.
- Forecasts of the outcome of the counselee's course of action.
- Assistance to the counselee in working out of solution of his problem.
- Follow up work.

45. Write the difference between guidance & Counselling?

Guidance	Counseling
Guidance is a process, which helps an individual to develop his personality fully and enables to serve the society to the best of his capabilities and talents.	Counseling is a series of direct contacts with the individual which aims to offer him assistance in changing his attitudes and behaviors.
Guidance is preventive.	Counseling is therapeutic
Guidance may be given any normal set up	Counseling requires a special set up
Decision making operates at intellectual level	Decision making operates at emotional level
It helps in promoting individual development	It helps in preventing future problem

46. What are the range of skills required for effective Counselling?

- Active Counselling
- Respecting
- Ientification
- Questioning

47. Write the basis of counselling and guidance.
- Individual basis
- Social basis

48. What are the steps of social basis?
Proper utilization of human resources
Family life betterment
Good citizenship.

49. What are the attributes of a counselling?
- Pertaining attributes
- Inter training attributes

50. Write two needs of a counsellor?
- An interested information adopted to an individual problem.
- He should posses the wide knowledge of the world and its basis.

51. Expand 'GATHER'.
G – Greet the client
A – Ask the client about themselves
T – **Tell** client or give the information of coping mechanisms
H – Help the client
E – Explain how to use a method.
R – Return for follow up.

52. Expand 'CLEAR'.
C – Clarify
L – Listen
E – Encourage
A – Acknowledge
R – Reflect and respect

53. Expand 'ROLES'.
R – Relax
O – Open and approachable.
L – Lean towards client
E – Eye contact
S – Smile and sit comfortably.

54. What are the types of counselling?
- Directive Counselling
- Nondirective Counselling
- Short term Counselling
- Long term Counselling

55. What are the types of interview?
- Introductory interview
- Fact finding interview
- Informative interview
- Therapeutic interview

56. What are the phases of interview?
- Preparation
- The process
- Interpretation

57. What are the types of case study?
- Formal case study
- Informal case study
- Descriptive case study
- Historical case study

58. List the ingredients of Counselling service.
- Planning service
- Placement service
- Follow up service
- Research and evaluation.

59. What are the problems in guidance and Counselling?
- Resistance to Counselling
- Counselee with different cultures
- Counsellor burn out.
- Lack of physical facilities.

60. What are the steps in counselling?
- Analysis
- Synthesis
- Diagnosis
- Prognosis
- Counselling
- Follow up

Test Series V

1. **Define education.**
Education is the natural, harmonious and progressive development of man's innate powers-Pestalozzi. Mahatama Gandhi once said Education is the all round drawing out of the best in child and man; body, mind and spirit.

2. **Discuss the functions of education.**
To complete the socialization process, to transmit the cultural heritage, formation of social personality, reformation of attitude, education for occupational placement, an instrument for livelihood, conferring the status, education encourages the spirit of competition, education trains in skills that one required by the economy, fosters participants democracy, education imparts values, education act as integrative force, values and orientation which are specific to certain professions are also provided by education.

3. **Write aims of education?**
Utilitarian aims are vocational, intellectual, citizenship, physical health and wellbeing, character development, moral development, education for leisure, self realization, mental and emotional development, autonomous development, self education, international understanding, homogeneous development.

4. **Define the types of education.**
Formal: Formal education is based on certain rules, customs and procedure.
Informal education: Is not systematically planned.
Non-formal education: Non formal education adopts a midway between formal & informal types of education. Eg. Correspondence education

5. **Define nursing education.**
Nursing education is a professional education which is consciously and systematically planned and implemented through instruction and discipline and aims the harmonious development of the physical, intellectual, social, emotional, spiritual and aesthetic powers or abilities of the student in order to render professional nursing service to people of all ages, in all phases of health and illness in a variety of settings in the best or highest possible manner.

6. **Define philosophy.**
Philosophy is an attempt to think truly about human experience or to make our

whole experience intelligible-Brightman Philosophy is increasing effort to discern the general truth that lies behind the particular facts discern also the reality that lies behind appearances-Raymonds.

7. **List down the traditional philosophies.**
   - Idealism,
   - Naturalism,
   - Pragmatism,
   - Realism
8. **List down the modern philosophies.**
   - Theistic realism,
   - Humanistic extentialism,
   - Eclectism.
9. **List down the principles of teaching.**
   Principle of motivation, principle of activity, teacher should arouse interest in students, there should be well defined objectives, principles of individual difference, principle of creativity, principles of selection, principles of division, principle of revision and practice, principle of correlation, principle of connecting with life.
10. **List the maxims of teaching.**
    Maxims of teaching are accepted truth or general rule of conduct or the laws which one essentially to be followed by the teacher while teaching.
    - Proceed from known to unknown
    - Proceed from concrete to abstract
    - Proceed from simple to complex
    - Proceed from easy to more difficult
    - Proceed inductively
    - Proceed from general to specific
    - Proceed from indefinite to definite
    - Proceed from empirical to rational
    - Proceed from whole to parts
    - Proceed from analysis to synthesis
    - Proceed from overview to details
    - From observation to reasoning
    - Proceed from psychological to logical.
11. **List the characteristics of learning.**
    Learning is growth, learning is adjustment, learning is organizing experience, learning is purposeful, learning is intelligent, learning is active, learning is both individual and social, learning affects the conduct of the learner, learning take place through trial and error, and learning depends upon insight.
12. **Enumerate the domains of learning.**
    Cognitive domain is concerned with information and knowledge, concepts, analysis, evaluation, synthesis and decision making belongs to the cognitive domain.
    Conative domain comprises of motor activities guided by human mind, manipulative skills, and operation of equipment are examples of psychomotor domain.
    The affective domain includes attitudes, values and concern for others.
13. **List the principles of education.**
    - Education is a continuous reorganization and integration of activities.
    - Education is both conservative and progressive.
    - Education is a psychological, sociological process.
    - Education is a process of self realization.
    - Education must be life long process.

Test Series VI

1. **Define teaching.**
   Teaching is the stimulation, guidance, direction and encouragement of learning. Teaching is a matter of helping the child to respond to his environment in an effective manner. The teacher simplifies the technique, modifies the environment, help the children to adjust, to strengthen the knowledge and helps them to develop beginning skills, abilities and knowledge.-Burton
2. **Define clinical teaching.**
   The clinical teaching is a type of group conference in which a patient or patients is (are) observed and studied, discussed, demonstrated and directed towards the improvement of nursing care.
3. **List out the types of clinical experiences and define any one.**
   Clinical experiences are divided into
   - Laboratory experiences
   - Supervised nursing care practice
   - Internship

   Definition of laboratory experiences:
   Students will learn the skills in laboratory situation on dummy or doll under strict supervision under guidance of clinical experts in specific field, the experience will be selected according to the curriculum.
4. **Write any purpose of clinical teaching.**
   - To provide individualized care in a systematic, holistic approach.
   - To develop cognitive, conative, affective and psychomotor skills.
   - To develop high technical competent skills
   - To practice various procedure.
5. **What are the methods of teaching in clinical area?**
   - Conferences
   - Bedside clinic
   - Nursing rounds
   - Ward class
   - Case method
   - Assignment
   - Brain storming method
   - Group discussion
   - Demonstration method
   - Laboratory method
   - Process recording
6. **Mention the types of conferences.**
   1) Group conference
   2) Nursing care conference
   3) Individual conference
   4) Team conference
   5) Staff conference

7. **Write three purpose of bedside clinic.**
To provide a learning experience for nursing student to collect information about the patient with act & skill.
To improve the students ability to solve nursing problems by detailed study & analysis of nursing situation
It helps the student to do nursing observation in an organized systematic way.

8. **What are the types of assignment?**
1) Preparatory assignments
2) Study assignments
3) Revision assignments
4) Remedial assignments

9. **Write some principles of assignment planning.**
a) It should correlate with previous experience.
b) It should motivate the students
c) It should challenge not threaten

10. **What are the outcomes of group discussions?**
- Increases knowledge
- Increased intellectual abilities & skills
- Increased interests

11. **Write one essential characteristic of good demonstration.**
The demonstrator should understand the entire procedure before attempting to perform for others, this sometimes necessitates review before performance.

12. **What are the techniques used in laboratory method?**
- Introducing phase
- Work period
- Culminating activities

13. **Define process recording.**
Process recording is an exact written report of the conversation between the nurse and patient during the time that they were together.

14. **List out the uses of process recording.**
- Teaching tool
- Self-evaluation tool
- Therapeutic tool

15. **What are phases of process recording?**
a) Preparing the student for process recording
b) Recording nurse patient interactions
c) Evaluating the nurse patient interactions

16. **List down some of the functions of the clinical instructor.**
- Set the objectives, standards for practice
- Develop evaluation tools
- Should take permission of the institution
- Prepare master rotation plan
- Set up the clinical area in an ideal manner.

17. **Write any five qualities of a clinical instructor.**
- Good observer
- Cheerful
- Open minded
- Listener
- Good discriminating power

18. **Write any four principles of clinical teaching.**
- Clinical teaching is a vital and irreplaceable component in preparing the nursing students for professional practice
- Clinical education should reflect the nature of professional practice
- Clinical teaching is important than class room teaching.
- The nursing student in the clinical setting is a learner, not a nurse.

19. **What are the purposes of group conference?**
- To set objectives and criteria for nurs-

ing care
- To plan methods for improving care
- To solve problems which interfere with good nursing care

20. Define group conference.

A conference is the act of consulting together, and coming together of two or more individuals in a formal meeting for the purpose of giving or exchanging ideas. It involves a two way flow of conversation.

21. Write any two purposes of nursing care conference.

- To portray the nursing problems typically associated with a particular disease with such factors as social, age or ethical background and to picture the related nursing care with a specific individual.
- To learn ways to help clients, identify their needs and solve their own problems.

22. What are types of nursing rounds?

1) Information giving rounds
2) Instructional rounds
3) Problem solving rounds

23. Define simulations.

According to international directory of education, simulation is a teaching technique used particularly in management education and training in, within a 'reel situation and values are simulated by substitute displaying similar characteristics.

24. Name types of simulation.

- Simulation exercise
- Simulation game
- Role playing

25. Write down the purpose of simulation.

- Help the students practice decision making and problem solving skills, and to develop human interaction abilities in a controlled and safe setting.
- Provide a chance to apply principles & theories.
- The knowledge gained through simulation can be easily transferred to the real patient care setting.
- Student achieves cognitive, affective & psychomotor outcomes

26. Define micro teaching.

According to Bush "micro teaching is a teacher to apply clearly defined teaching skills, to carefully prepared class one in a planned series of five to ten minutes, encounter with a small group of real students of ten with an opportunity to observe the result on video tape".

27. Write the phases of micro teaching.

a) Knowledge acquisition phase
b) Skill acquisition phase
c) Transfer phase

28. Define programmed instruction.

Programmed instruction is a progressively monitored, step by step teaching method, employing small units of information or learning material and frequent testing, whereby student must complete or pass one stage before moving on to the next. Also called as programmed learning.

29. List down the principles of programmed instruction.

a) Objective specification
b) Frequent testing
c) Self-facing
d) Principle of active responding
e) Student testing

30. Write down the types of programming.

a) The linear
b) The bean
c) The mathematics
d) Adjusts
e) Computer generated instruction

31. Define computer assisted learning.

It is an approach to language teaching &learning in which computer technology is used as an aid to the presentation, reinforcement & assessment of material to be learned. Usually including a sustainable interactive element.

32. List down the methods used in computer assisted learning.

1) Video tutorials
2) Demonstration
3) Workshops (on site learning workshop)

33. Define workshop.

A workshop is a room or building which provides both the area and tools that may be required for the manufacture or repair of manufactured goods.

34. Define field trip.

A field trip is a visit especially planned for its possible contribution to the objectives of the curriculum, course, project lesson or other list of instructions.

35. Write down the steps in organizing field trip knowledge.

1) report
2) Objectives
3) Time & transportation
4) Preparation of students
5) Supervision

36. List down the disadvantage of field trip.

1) Time consuming
2) Effective observation become difficult
3) Careful planning is needed
4) Cooperation, coordination of various agencies required.

37. Define self instructional model.

A self instruction model is to teach system-based, practice based learning and improvement. Self instruction is the designation of materials or programs that are designed to provide independent learning; this is in other words means to teach oneself or to learn by oneself without obtaining the assistance from others

38. Write down the types of self instructional method.

- Distance education or distance learning
- Multimedia learning
- E learning
- M learning

39. Write down the advantages of computer assisted instruction.

- A lot of data can be stored
- Learners responses and the feedback can be easily obtained
- Performance & marks are easily visible

40. Define exhibition.

An exhibition, in the most general sense, is an organized presentation and display of a selection of items. In practice, exhibitions usually occur within museums, galleries, exhibition halls, and World's Fairs. Exhibitions can include many things such as art in both major museums and smaller galleries, interpretive exhibitions, natural history museums and history museums, and also varieties such as more commercially focused exhibitions and trade fairs.

41. List the steps in organizing exhibition.

- Determine the exhibition theme
- Choose a data
- Seek out supplemental funding
- Plan the collection of material
- Create informational labels for all the works.
- Identify the most important piece to illustrate the exhibits theme
- Plan the publicity program
- Supervise the hanging and placements of the work

42. List down the skills for micro teaching.

- Skill of probing questions
- Skill of explaining
- Skill of illustration with example
- Skill of reinforceement
- Skill of stimulus variation

43. Define lecture method.

"Lecture is a teaching activity whereby the teacher presents the content in a comprehensible manner by explaining the facts, principles and relationships, during which the teacher is expected to elicit student participation by employing appropriate techniques"

44. State lecturing techniques.

- Voluntary dissemination of information or spontaneity
- Voice gradation and voice quality
- Adequate pacing
- Proper body language
- Control annoying mannerisms
- Judicious use of audio-visual aids
- Simple plan & key points
- Elicit feedback from students
- Providing further clarification
- Time management

45. Define demonstration.

"Demonstration is a method of teaching by exhibition and explanation combined to illustrate a procedure or experiments'"

46. List the phases of demonstration.

- Planning & preparation phase: In the planning and preparation phase
- Teacher prepares herself, arranges necessary articles and creates a conducive learning environment suitable to number of students.
- Performance phase: In this phase, teacher performs the demonstration, throughout this phase she has to maintain positive approach by telling "what to do "rather "what no to do". She exhibit coordination of head, heart & hand.
- Evaluation phase: Evaluation is done mainly through return demonstration & asking thought provoking questions

47. State the purpose of discussion.

- To teach context specific interpretation and application of principles, theories and concepts:
- Assist students to develop, express and validate their opinions' or beliefs regarding legal, ethical and controversial issues in nursing
- To clarify information and concepts
- To share information
- To foster democratic values
- To develop team building and social skills
- Development of right attitudes
- To develop problem solving skills as a group
- To arouse students interest

48. State advantages & disadvantages of discussion method.

Advantages:

- Discussion is an excellent student centered method, active participation also promotes presentation & recalling abilities of students
- Acceptance of students' opinion.

Disadvantages:

- Difficult to complete within allotted time period
- Needs adequate preparation of students. If not prepared becomes less effective.
- Less effective if number of student exceeds 20.

49. Mention types of seminar.

Based on the level of organization, seminar can be classified into:

- **Mini seminar** – Conducted in class room
- **Main seminar** – Organized at department or institutional level.
- **National & international seminar** – Conducted at national & international level.

50. Mention the personnel involved in seminar.

Organizers, chairperson, speakers & participants

Organizer:

- Selects the topic
- Selects the chair person
- Set objectives and coordinate the full seminar

Chairperson:

- Introduces the topic & justifies the selection by stating its importance.
- Once speaker completes his speech, gives a brief summary of it & involves next speaker.

Speaker:

- Prepare & hand over study material to organizer. Expected to present relevant information in an interesting and comprehensible manner.

Participants:

- Utilize the discussion session by asking questions, seeking clarification & expressing their view points.

51. Define symposium.

Symposium is a form of discussion in which different viewpoints or opinions regarding the single aspect or component of a topic are discussed under the guidance of chairperson.

52. List difference between seminar & symposium.

	Seminar	Symposium
1.	Topics are related to recent trends and development in nursing.	Topics are related to controversial issues in nursing.
2.	Multiple aspects of topic is discussed.	single aspect of topic is discussed
3.	Chair person has to exert less control	chair person has to exert more control
4.	Less time for discussion involving participants	more time for discussion involving participants
5.	Less preparation from side of participants.	more preparation from side of participants.

53. Define role-playing.

Role playing is a form of drama in which learners spontaneously act out roles in an interaction involving problems or challenges in human relations for subsequent discussion by the whole class.

54. Define problem based learning.

"The basic outline of PBL process is encountering the problem first, problem solving with clinical skills and identifying learning needs in an interactive process of self study, applying new gained knowledge to the problem and summarizing what has been learned" -Barrows

55. Write the advantages of PBL.

- Emphasis on measuring, not facts

- Increased self direction
- Higher comprehension and better skill development
- Interpersonal skills and team work
- Self motivated attitude
- Facilitator student relationship

56. Write the steps in PBL.

Step1: The problem is presented to the group, terms are reviewed & hypothesis generated. The student will be expected to solve the problem.

Step2: Learning issues &independent sources are identified.

Step3: Iinformation gathering & independent study occur.

Step4: The knowledge acquired is discussed & debated critically.

Step5: Knowledge is applied to problem in a practical way.

Step6: Reflection on control & process learning occur.

57. Define panel discussion.

Panel is a discussion in which a few persons carry on a conversation in front of an audience. When the group is too large to work effectively through the usual round table procedure.

58. Write the technique of panel discussion.

The chairman begins the panel discussion by exploring the whole proceedings.

First, the members of panel are introduced by name & back ground of experience. The topic is announced & limits of the discussion are started. The chairman may start the procedure, Introduce each participant briefly, mentioning only a relevant facts about her experience or involvement related to the topic and making a comment or two or by directing a question to a particular person. The chairman encourage the different opinion, a general summary before discussion is opened to audience

59. Define project method.

"A project is a problematic act carried to completion its natural setting" -Stevenson

"A whole-hearted purposeful activity proceeding in a social environment".

60. List the types of projects.

Dr.Kilpatrick has suggested 4 types

Producer type: In which pupils are getting to do something. E.g.: model of house.

Consumer type: Projects in which pupils are getting the experience and are enjoying, engaged in consumer type.

Problem type: Project in which a solution to a problem is to be found out.

Drill type: An activity once performed, is repeated to acquire greater skill e.g.: swimming, singing.

61. Mention five merits of project method.

- Follows psychological laws of learning
  - -law of readiness
  - -law of exercise
  - -law of effect
- Gives freedom to pupils
- Suited to psychological concept of maturation
- Social values derived
- Training for social adjustments.

62. List the disadvantages of role play.

- Role play is a mean not an end
- Require guidance and leadership
- Participants may feel threatened
- Used as an education technique, not as a therapeutic one.
- Time consuming in developing group readiness.
- Limited only by teachers ingenuity.

Test Series VII

1. Define AV aids.

An audio visual aids is an instruction device in which the message can be heard as well as seen. It helps in the process of learning. i.e. motivation, clarification and stimulation.

2. List the purposes of AV aids.

Quicken the phase of learning.
Improves and make teaching effective.
Saves time and energy.
Increases and retain attention and concentration
Makes learning interesting and profitable.

3. Mention the principles to be followed in using AV aids.

- AV aids materials should function as an integral part of educational programme.
- AV aids should be centralized, under specification, direction and leadership in education program.
- AV education program should be flexible.

4. Clarify AV aids.

- Auditory aids
  Radio & Recording
- Visual aids
  Projected Non projected
  Over head projector 3D materials
- Audio visual aids e.g. television
- Aid through activity e.g. field trip
- Traditional media: dramas.

5. Explain the sources of audio visual aids.

- Government
- Educational institution
- Professional organization
- Non government organization.
- Commercial producers of educations material.

6. List the factors influencing A.V aids:

- The objectives of training programme.
- The nature of subject matter being taught
- Nature of audience
- Availability of cost.

7. What are graphic materials?

It is a combination of graphic and pictorial material designed for orderly and logical visualizing of relationships between key facts and ideas.

It includes: Graphs, charts, maps, diagrams.

8. Specify the essential qualities of a model.

- Accuracy
- Simplicity
- Clarity
- Reliability
- Ingenuity

- Usefullness

9. What are dimensional aids?
- Objects
- Specimen
- Models
- Puppets

10. List the types of models.
- Scale model
- Simplified model
- Working model
- Cross section model

11. Mention the types of chalk board.
- Photographs
- Cutout illustrations
- Publications
- Drawing
- Specimen

12. Enlist the types of bulletin board.
- Flannel board/felt board
- Magnetic board
- Fixed type
- Folded type.

13. Write the rules to prepare posters.
- Use bold letters (20"*30").
- Use pleasing colours.
- Tell message in a single glance.
- To promote one point.

14. List the types of charts.
- Narrative chart
- Cause and effect chart
- Chain chart
- Evolution chart
- Strip tear chart
- Pull charts.

15. Define pamphlets.

Pamphlets can be folded into two, three or five, the matter will be printed either single side or both sides.

16. Define flannel/felt board.

The rigid material covered with flannel cloth/felt sheet/wool/cotton/paper reed cloth. The items to be displayed should have flannel or sand paper pasted on reverse side.

17. Specify the effective use of AV aids.
- Planning.
- Preparation
- Presentation
- Evaluation.

18. Describe visual aids.

Projected – Over head projector

Non projected aids – Photographs/illustration/backboard

19. List the principles in use of bulletin board.
- The appearance of them must be neat, orderly and attractive manner.
- Material should be changed frequently and systematically to encourage interest.
- Crowding of display material should be avoided.

20. Mention the types of recording.
1) Phonograph recording
2) Wire recording
3) Tape recording

21. List the purposes of clinical teaching.
- To provide individualized care in a systematic, holistic approach
- To develop high technical competent skills
- To practice various procedure
- To conduct research
- To collect & analyze the data.

22. What is the meaning of group discussion?

A co-operative, problem solving activity which seeks a consensus regarding the solution of a problem

23. What is role play?

An educational technique in which people spontaneously act out problems of human relation and analyze the enactment with the help of other role players and observers.

24. Mention the steps of role playing.

- Select the problem for role playing
- Set up the role playing scene
- Getting underway in role playing
- The part the group plays
- Cutting the role playing
- The role playing is cut
- The audience expressing ideas

25. Mention 3 types of programming.

- The linear
- The branching
- The mathematics

26. Mention the steps in programme writing.

- Preparation
- Programme writing
- Try out & revision

27. What is the disadvantage of symposium?

- Lack of time
- Inadequate opportunity for all the students to participate actively
- Time is limited to 15 to 20 min
- Audience participation is limited

28. What is panel discussion?

Panel is a discussion in which a few person carry on a conversation in front of an audience when the group is too large to work effectively through the usual round table procedure

29. List 4 types of puppet? Mention their use?

- Finger puppet
- Hand puppet
- Rod puppet
- Marionette (String puppet)

Uses:

- Effective listening skills
- Group co-operation
- Co-operation and self control
- Understand the subject content

30. Define maps and list types of maps.

Maps are graphic representation of the earth's surface or portions of it as formed as maps.

Types:

- Relief maps
- Historical maps
- Distinction maps
- Geographical maps

31. What are the elements of cartoon?

- Personalized humour
- Fun

32. Define over-head projector?

Overhead projector is a device for projecting a matter, which is written or drawn on transparent sheet of acetate on to a screen.

33. What are the advantages of OHP?

- If permits the teacher to stand in front of the class while the projector is focusing the matter.
- concepts can be illustrated
- It can be used well in a fairly well-lighted room.
- Transparencies can be changed easily and quickly.

34. What are audio devices?

Radio, tape recording, FM.

35. What are the characteristics of audio experience?

- Immediacy
- Emotional
- Audible
- Congruent of time & space
- One way communication

Test Series VIII

1. **Define attitude scale.**

   An attitude scale attempts to obtain a precise measure of the eternity of people's attitudes. The accuracy of the measurement can be increased by using many items that are all related to the same issue.

2. **List down any two uses of attitude scales.**
   - To measure the social attitudes.
   - Some relevant and indirect statements will be used to reveal the attitude.
   - The scale also specifies the crucial shades of opinion.

3. **Mention the types of attitude scales.**
   - Differential scale (LL thurstone scale)
   - Point scale
   - Summated (Likert) scale.
   - Cumulative scale/Bogadus social distance scale.

4. **Explain the methods used in point scale.**

   Method-1.
   - Select the words which will give the opinion
   - The respondent is to cross out every word.
   - The attitude of a respondent is known by calculating the numbers of words crossed.
   - One point is given to each agreement or disagreement whichever is to be chosen.

   Method-2
   - Two sets of words indicating both favourable and unfavourable opinions are given. The unfavourable opinions are crossed and favourable items may be left unscored.

5. **What are the uses of likert scale over the thurstone scale?**
   - The method of construction of likert scale is less cumbersome.
   - It supplies more precise and definite response towards an issue.
   - The likert scale permits the revelation of several 5 degrees of agreement or disagreement but thurstone scale is based on only two alternative responses.

6. **List the deficits in likert type scale.**

   The judgement on the basis of total score is estimated by calculating the mean or median. The scores on the likert type scale may be helpful for making an ordering of the people.

   There is no objective basis for expressing different degrees of agreement or disagreement.

7. **List down the methods of assessing at-**

titude.

Interview, assignments, communicative records, anecdotal Records, observation during performance, critical incident technique, discussion.

8. Define scale.

A scale is a continuum intermediate points in-between these two terms.

9. List down any two difficulties in scaling.

- It is not possible to assess the validity directly.
- Social phenomena are complex and qualitative in nature.
- No universal recognized measuring tool.
- The social phenomena cannot be experimented in a controlled way.

10. List down the types of scales.

- Nominal scale
- Ordinal scale
- Interval scale/cardinal scale.
- Ratio scale
- Rating scales.

11. Define teaching method?

Teaching method is the simulation, guidance, direction and encouragement for learning.

12. Mention some of the objectives of methods of teaching.

- Aim at developing, "love for work".
- Develops the capacity for clear thinking.
- Expands student's interest.
- Provides opportunities to pupils to apply practically the knowledge and skill acquired by them.
- General support of the profession.

13. List down classification of teaching methods.

- Inspirational methods
- Expository methods
- Natural learning method
- Individualized method
- Encounter method
- Discovery method
- Group methods.

14. What is the purpose of clinical teaching?

- To provide individualized care in a systematic, holistic approach.
- To develop high technical completed skills.
- To practice various procedures.
- To collect and analyze the data.
- To conduct research.
- To maintain high standard of nursing practice.
- To develop cognitive, conative, affective and psychomotor skills.

15. What are nursing rounds?

A small group of the staff members not more than five and a leader or teacher visit, the bedside of clients. Nursing superintendents, ward sisters taking rounds of the hospital wards. It helps the nursing members know about all the patients in the wards, their problems and ways of solving. It is an extension of the clinic method.

16. What is care analysis?

A concrete care for analysis and discussion by a group of students under the leadership of the instructor, sufficient information is presented to the students to make judgement of problem or situation in care.

17. Write the types of assignments.

- Patient assignment
- Work assignment
- Student assignment
- Special assignment
- Functional assignment
- Combination assignment

- Team assignment
- Case method assignment

18. Define checklist.

A list of items with appropriate columns is made, it can be checked off by the observer. Checklist may only provide for yes or no responses. To assure no task is left un answered, diagnosis or grading check lists will be used.

19. Write advantage of demonstration method.

- The teacher is present
- Gives a feeling of security
- Develops the quality of observation
- Ensures close contact with concrete problems.
- Facilitates the acquisition of practical, intellectual and communication skills.
- Presents reality, not substitutes
- Enables logical step by step presentation.
- Is attention catching
- Demonstrates the right way of doing a computer task.
- Presented facing the audience.
- Makes it possible to ask questions
- Limits damage to equipment and material when students do practical work afterwards.

20. Define programmed instruction.

It is a kind of learning in which a "program" takes the place of a tutor for the student and leads him through a set of frames of specified behaviours designed and sequenced to make it more probable that will behave in a given desired way [Kochhar s.k.S.K 1992].

21. Write the five 'R' of micro-teaching.

- Recording
- Reviewing
- Responding
- Refining
- Re-doing

22. What is process recording?

An exact written report of the conversation between the nurse and the patient during the time they were together, and a record of the nurses feelings about what was going on at the time, and as far as possible 'how the patient said what he did' -Hudson.

23. State the types of nursing audit.

- Patient questionnaire
- Bedside chart review
- Retrospective chart review
- Concurrent chart review.

24. What is panel discussion?

Panel is a discussion in which a few persons carry on a conversation in front of an audience. When the group is too large to work effectively through the usual round-table procedure.

25. Write purpose of symposium technique?

- To investigate a problem from several points of view.
- To boost the students ability to speak in a group.
- To make the students to study independently.

26. Define workshop?

A group of individuals who work together the solution of problems in a given subject matter field during a specific period of time.

27. What is team teaching?

A type of instructional organization, involving teaching personnel and the students and the students assigned to them, in which two or more teachers are given responsibility working together, for all or significant part of the instruction of the same groups of students.

28. Mention the guiding principles of team teaching.

- Size and composition
- Time factor
- Learning environment
- Duties assigned to teachers should be appropriate.
- Level of instruction
- Supervision.

29. Write the phase of process recording.

1) Preparing the student for process recording
2) Recording nurse-patient interaction
3) Evaluating the nurse-patient interaction.

30. What is laboratory method?

Laboratory method is a procedure involving first hand experience with primary source materials, through which the student can acquire psychomotor as well as mental skills.

Test Series IX

1. **Define health behaviour.**
   Behavior that promote health, prevent illness and help in the cure of and rehabilitation of sick people.
2. **Mention phases of change in behaviour.**
   - Awareness
   - Interest
   - Evaluation
   - Trial
   - Adoption
   - Conviction
3. **Write the dynamics of the behavioural change cycle.**
   - Pre contemplative
   - Contemplative
   - Preparing
   - Action
   - Maintaining
   - Termination
4. **Write the characteristics of effective health education.**
   - Promotes actions
   - Builds on ideas, concepts and practices that people already have.
   - Repeats and reinforces information overtime.
   - Uses existing channels of communication skills.
   - Entertains and attracts the attention of the communication.
   - Uses clear, simple language.
   - Uses demonstrations to show the benefits of adopting practices.
5. **Write the methods of health education.**
   - Lecture
   - Group discussion
   - Demonstration
   - Panel discussion
   - Symposium
   - Workshop
   - Role playing
   - Programmed instruction
   - Simulation exercises.
6. **List the roles of community health nurse in health education process.**
   - She is an educator, as well as learner
   - An organizer and counsellor
   - A liaison between the community, home, hospital and other members of the team.
7. **Mention the behaviours that affect health.**
   Alcohol, smoking, less physical activity, nutrition, accidents.
8. **Write principles of health education.**
   - Credibility

- Interest
- Participation
- Motivation
- Comprehension
- Reinforcement
- Learning by doing
- Known to unknown
- Setting an example
- Good human relation
- Feedback
- Leaders.

9. **What are approaches to health education?**
   - Regulator approach (managed prevention)
   - Service approach
   - Health education approach
   - Primary health care approach

Test Series X

1. **Define health education.**
   Health education is a process which affects changes in the health practices of people and in the knowledge and attitudes related to such changes.
2. **What are objectives of health education?**
   - Informing people
   - Motivating people
   - Guiding into action.
3. **What are the principles in planning health promotion?**
   - Health promotion involves the population as a whole in the context of everyday life, rather than focusing on people at risk for specific diseases.
   - Health promotion is directed towards actions on the determinants causes of health.
   - Health promotion combines diverse but complementary methods.
   - Health promotion aims particularly at effective public participation.
4. **What are the changes that occur by planning health education?**
   Learning, perception, knowledge, attitude, motivation decision, behavior, propaganda are the some of the changes occurred by planning health education.
5. **List down the steps for a group approach.**
   Introduction
   Modification of attitude & behavior.
   Communication.
6. **What are the levels of health education?**
   - Community approach
   - Individual approach
   - Group approach
   - Family approach
7. **List functions of health education planning.**
   - To train key health & community welfare works in health education.
   - To prepare & produce health education material, both printed & audio visual, for the general public & for health training purposes.
8. **Where central training institutes located?**
   - National Institute of Health & Family Welfare, New Delhi.
   - Central Health Education Bureau, New Delhi.
   - All India Institute of Hygiene & Public Health, Kolkata
   - Family Welfare Training and Research Centre, Mumbai.
   - Rural Health & Family Welfare Training Centre. Gandhigtron, TN.

9. How knowledge is perceived?

It is the collection and storage of information (or) experience (i.e. knowledge = preparation + storage information in the brain).

10. What are the types mass media?

- Television
- Radio
- Internet
- Newspapers
- Printed materials
- Direct mailing
- Posters, bill boards and signs
- Health museums and exhibitions
- Folk media

11. Enlist two points using a television programme as classroom instructional aid.

- Collect other instructional materials that relate to the programme which you wish students to watch in the classroom
- Motivate students to watch the program critically and for specific details.

12. Enlist the advantages of educational television programme.

- It can receive the past events and happenings.
- The television can work as a powerful medium of mass education.

13. Describe radio.

The radio has a broad audience than T.V it is a cheaper, health workers may identify and discuss health issues leading to increased general awareness.

14. Write about Internet.

This new means of computer based communication system has opened vast capability of transfer of knowledge and has made it possible to get into direct and instant communication across the world.

15. Enumerate the limitations of newspapers.

Newspapers have limitation of having low readership because of illiteracy.

16. List any 4 printed materials.

Magazines, pamphlets, booklets, handouts.

17. Write about direct mapling.

This is new innovation in health communication. The intention is to reach the remote areas of the country with printed word.

18. What are the advantages of health museums and exhibitions?

- It can attract large numbers of people.
- By presenting a variety of ideas, they do increase knowledge and awareness.

19. Write the meaning of folk media.

Folk media is keerthan, katha, folksongs, dances and dramas and puppet shows which have roots in our culture.

20. Define communication.

It is a process by which meaning or thoughts are exchanged between individuals through the mutually understood language or symbol.

21. Write the objectives of communication.

• To be received • To be understood
• To be accepted • To get action

22. What are the types of communications?

- Verbal Communication
- Non Verbal Communication
- Written Communication

23. What are the components of communication?

• Source (sender) • Receiver (audience
• Message (content) • Channels (medium)
• Feedback (effect).

24. Mention the barriers of communication.

Physiological – Hearing & expression difficulties

Psychological – Emotional disturbances, levels of intelligence, language or comprehension difficulties.

Environmental – Noise

25. Contents of health education.

- Human biology • Nutrition • Hygiene
- Family health • Disease prevention and control • Mental health • Prevention of accidents • Use of health services.

26. Write any four communication function.

- Information • Education • Motivation
- Counselling

27. List down the four responsibilities of counsellor.

- To communicate information.
- To gain the trust of the people
- To help people reduce or resolve their problems.
- To listen sympathetically to people who are anxious, distressed

28. List any two characteristics of right kind of information.

- Increase awareness at the people
- Brings changes in health seeking behaviour

29. Define persuasion.

A conscious attempt by one individual to change or influence the general benefits, values and behavior of another individuals, or group of individuals in some desired way.

MEDICAL SURGICAL NURSING-I

INTRODUCTION

The fundamental basis of nursing practice is called nursing process, which includes problem solving and decision making. It is accepted as a tool and methodology applicable to the nursing profession. Nursing process is a deliberate rational approach to discharge nursing care in an effective and systematic manner.

Critical thinking

Excellence in the delivery of nursing requires good thinking. Every day nurses make many decisions that affect the care of their patients. For those to be effective, the thinking behind them must be sound. Critical thinking is the use of cognitive skills or strategies that increase the probability of a desirable outcome. (Halpern).

Evidence based practice

It is a systematic process that employs current evidence to make decisions about patient care. It includes evaluation of the quality and applicability of existing research, patient preferences, costs, clinical expertise and clinical settings. Evidence gives assurance that nursing practice will be effective.

Issues in nursing practice

The nurse is guided by the law and standards set forth by the profession. A professional code of ethics provides a framework. Some of the major ethical obligations of nursing practice are addressed in the code of ethics. Some of the terms in the code of ethics include fidelity, veracity, integrity, compassion, discernment, trustworthiness and respectfulness.

Multidimensional role of Medical Surgical Nursing

Nurses specializing in Medical Surgical Nursing should have a broad knowledge of biological, psychological and social sciences because they are expected to cater to the needs of the patient. Roles of a nurse include critical thinking, care provider, care planner, care coordinator, educator, researcher, advocate etc.

Special care units

Medical/ surgical intensive care units

Cardiac intensive care units

Burns care unit

Trauma care unit

Outpatient care unit and other special care units like dialysis care unit etc.

Fluid and electrolyte, acid base imbalance

Fluids are located in various compartments within the body. Fluid imbalances are common in clinical settings. Patients in the hospital are at the highest risk of life threatening complications that result from excess or deficit of fluid called dehydration or over hydration. At times patients may also experience problems because of too much or too little electrolytes. Acid base imbalances are caused by number of acute and chronic illnesses or conditions.

Nutritional imbalances

If the diet is deficient of any nutrients, malnutrition may results and an individual may suffer from physical and mental growth retardation. Nutritional disorders are categorized as under : Undernutrition, malnutrition, obesity, effect of natural toxins in food.

Disease concepts and disease prevention

Disease is state of abnormal bodily function. Major causes of disease are: Genetic error, trauma, microbial infections by pathogens, altered immunity, allergy and hypersensitivity, deficency diseases and idiopathic.

Classification of illness

Acute and sub acute, chronic, acute or chronic terminal illness.

References

1. Black, J.M., & Jacobs, E. M (1998). **Medical and Surgical Nursing, Clinical Management for Continuity of Care**. 5th ed. W.B. Saunders.
2. BT Basvanthappa, (2005) **Medical Surgical Nursing** 1st ed. Jaypee
3. Lewis, S. M., (2007). **Medical Surgical Nursing: Assessment & Management of Clinical Problems** 6th ed. Mosby.
4. Lippincott. (2008). **Manual of Nursing Practice** 8th ed. Williams & Wilkins publications.
5. Phipps etal. (2007). **Medical Surgical Nursing Health & Illness Perspective** 8th ed. Mosby publications.
6. Smelter, S. C., & Brenda, G.B (1992). **Brunner and Suddarth's Textbook of Medical Surgical Nursing** 7th ed. Lippincott.

Test Series I

1. **Define Illness.**
   Illness is a highly personal state in which the person's, physical, emotional, intellectual, social development or spiritual functioning is thought to be diminished. It is not synonymous with disease.
2. **List down the types of immunity.**
   Natural Immunity:
   It is a non specific immunity present at birth. It provides a non specific response to any foreign invader regardless of the invader's Composition.
   Acquired Immunity:
   Immunological responses acquired during life, but not present at birth usually develops as a result of prior exposure to an antigen through Immunization (Vaccination).
3. **Enumerate the types of pain.**
   - Somatic pain.
   - Visceral pain.
   - Centrally generated pain.
   - Peripherally generated pain.
4. **Write some nursing interventions to reduce fever.**
   - Exposure to cool air by an electric fan.
   - Administration of cool drinks.
   - Application of cold compress, ice bags.
   - Cold sponging and cold packs.
5. **Define acute illness.**
   Acute illness is typically characterized by severe symptoms of relatively short duration. The symptoms often appear abruptly and subside quickly & depending upon the cause. May or may not require intervention by health care professionals.
6. **Write the phases of wound healing.**
   - Inflammatory also called lag (exudative Phase) -- Duration: 1-4 days
   - Proliferative also called fibroblastic or connective tissue phase -- Duration: 5-20 days.
   - Maturation also called differentiation, resorptive
   - remodeling or plateau phase -- Duration: 21 days to months or years.
7. **Name the characteristics of pain.**
   - Pattern of pain.
   - Area of pain.
   - Intensity of pain.
   - Quality of pain.
   - Associated symptoms.
8. **Name the levels of unconsciousness.**
   - Alertness, oriented.
   - Lethargy, sleepy.

- Stupor.
- Semi-coma stage.
- Coma.

9. Define chronic illness.

It is defined as the one that lasts for an extended period, usually 6 months or longer and often for the person's life. It usually has a slow onset & often has periods of remissions & exacerbation, when the symptoms reappear.

10. What are the stages of illness?

- Symptom Experience.
- Assumption of the sick role.
- Medial Care contact.
- Dependent client role.
- Recovery or Rehabilitation.

11. List down the role of nurse in home health care.

- Home health nurses provide creative & adaptive care to the client.
- A holistic, non-judgemental & family centered philosophy is essential in the home care.
- A sincere commitment to health promotion & maintenance.
- Provide individualized care, promote independent of the client.

12. Define inflammation.

Inflammation is non specific response to an injury, meaning the same sequence of events occurs regardless of the cause. Inflammation brings fluid dissolved substances & the blood clots into the interstitial tissue.

13. Mention types of types of inflammation.

- Acute Inflammation: It is a short term reaction of the body to any tissue damage. It is immediate and usually lasts less than 1 to 2 week.
- Chronic Inflammation: It is slower in onset and lasts weeks to months or year.

14. Define infection.

Invasion and growth of the micro organism will lead to disease. Micro organism may be bacteria, viruses, fungi, protozoa or metazoan.

15. Write the six Steps in "the chain of infection".

- Etiologic agent (Micro organism).
- Reservoir (Source).
- Portal of exit from reservoir.
- Method of transmission.
- Portal of entry to the susceptible host.
- Susceptible host.

16. Define immunity.

The term "immunity" refers to the body's specific protective response to an invading foreign agent or organism.

17. What are the factors affecting wound healing process?

- Age of patient
- Hemorrhage
- Hypovolemia
- Edema
- Infection
- Oxygen deficit
- Inadequate dressing technique

18. What is edema?

Accumulation of fluid into the interstitial space is called edema.

19. What are causes of edema?

- Elevation of various hydrostatic pressure.
- Decrease in plasma osmotic pressure.
- Elevation of interstitial osmotic pressure.

20. List down the types of edema.

- Pitting edema.
- Non pitting edema.
- Facial edema.

- Lower limb edema.
- Pulmonary edema.

21. List the clinical manifestation of edema.
- Soft skin
- Increased body weight
- Fatigue
- Leg cramps
- Flabby muscle
- Paresthesia
- Decreased reflexes

22. Write some of the electrolyte imbalance.

Sodium imbalance.

Hyper natremia.

Hypo natremia.

Potassium imbalance

Hyperkalemia.

Hypokalemia.

Calcium imbalance

Hypercalcemia

Hypocalcemia.

23. Classify pain.
- Nociceptive pain
- Neuropathic pain.
- Acute and chronic pain.

24. List some drug for treatment of pain.

Non opioid:
- Acetaminophen.
- Aspirin.
- Ibuprofen.
- Diclofenac.

Opioids:
- Morphine
- Hydromorphone.
- Methadone
- Fentanyl

25. Define and list causes of incontinence.

Definition: Inability to voluntarily control discharge of urine.

Causes: Neurogenic bladder, bladder infection, injury to external sphincter.

26. List down some age related problems.
- Incontinence.
- Activity intolerance.
- Fatigue.
- Infertility.

27. Define osmosis.

Osmosis is the movement of water between two compartments separated by a semi permeable membrane. Water moves through the membrane from an area of low solute concentration to an area of high solute concentration.

28. What are the causes of hyponatremia?

Excessive sodium loss.

GI losses: diarrhoea, vomiting.

Renal losses: burns, wound drainage.

29. Define syncope.

Temporary loss of consciousness caused by a fall in blood pressure

30. Define fever or pyrexia.

Fever or pyrexia defined as a rise in the body temperature above 99° F.

31. What are the types of fever?
- Constant fever.
- Remittent fever.
- Relapsing fever.
- Rigor.
- Intermittent fever.

32. What are the biological theories?
- Crosslink theory.
- Free radical theory.
- Immunologic theory.
- Wear and tear theory.

33. What are factors helping in successful aging?
- Regular medical checkup.
- Adequate and appropriate treatment of diseases.
- Adequate nutrition.
- Provide adequate time for rest and sleep.

- Passive and active exercise.

34. Define septic shock.

Septic shock is the presence of sepsis with hypotension despite fluid resuscitation along with the presence of tissue perfusion abnormalities. It is systematic inflammatory response to suspected infection.

35. Define cardiogenic shock.

Cardiogenic shock occurs when either systolic or diastolic dysfunction of the pumping action of the heart result in compromised cardiac output. The heart inability to pump the blood forward is classified as systolic dysfunction.

36. Define anaphylactic shock.

Anaphylactic shock is an acute life threatening hypersensitive reaction to a sensitizing substance (drugs, chemicals, vaccine and food).

37. Define neurogenic shock.

Neurogenic shock is a hemodynamic phenomenon that can occur within 30 minute of a spinal cord injury at the fifth thoracic vertebra or above and lasts up to 6 weeks.

38. List down the signs and symptoms of hypokalemia and its treatment.

Signs anad symptoms: Muscle cramping, muscle fatigue, shallow respiration, diminished skeletal muscle activity, weak irregular pulse, dysrhythmias, orthostatic hypotension, neurologic changes, slowed GI motility and vomiting.

Treatment: Oral potassium supplement for mild to moderate hypokalemia, for severe hypokalemis-IV potassium is given wih IV fluids

39. What are the signs of hypocalcemia and its correction treatment?

Signs: Increased and irregular heart beat, mental status changes, hyperactive DTR, increased GI motility, Classic signs: Trousseaus sign, positive chovestek's sign.

Treatment: Oral calcium supplements with or without Vitamin-D, calcium rich diet. Severe hypocalcemia is corrected with IV calcium.

Test Series II

1. **Define dyspnea.**
   Dyspnea is a symptom common in many pulmonary and cardiac disorders, particularly when there is decreased lung compliance or increased airway resistance. (Difficult or labored breathing, shortness of breath).
2. **List out the causes for pulmonary edema.**
   - Heart failure.
   - Overhydration with intravenous fluids
   - Hypoalbuminemia, nephrotic syndrome, hepatic disease.
   - Respiratory distress syndrome.
   - Malignancies of the lymph system.
3. **Mention the steps in chest physiotherapy.**
   - Percussion
   - Vibration
   - Postural drainage
4. **What is meant by atelectasis?**
   It is a condition of the lungs characterized by collapsed, airless alveoli. The most common cause of atelectasis is airway obstruction that results from retained exudates and secretions.
5. **What are all the complications of TB?**
   - Miliary TB.
   - Pleural effusion and emphysema.
   - Tuberculosis pneumonia.
   - Other organ involvement (CNS, bone, and kidneys).
6. **What is cyanosis?**
   Cyanosis is a bluish discoloration of the skin due to deoxygenated hemoglobin in the blood. It appears when there is 5g/dl of deoxygenated haemoglobin.
7. **List out the clinical manifestations of pulmonary embolism.**
   - Dyspnea
   - Chest pain
   - Hemoptysis
   - Tachypnea, tachycardia.
   - Dependent oedema of the legs
8. **Define cystic fibrosis.**
   It is an autosomal recessive, multisystem disease characterized by altered function of the exocrine glands primarily involving the lungs, pancreas, and sweat glands.
9. **What is flial chest?**
   Flial chest results from multiple rib fractures causing an unstable chest wall with the paradoxical chest wall movement.
10. **Mention about diagnostic studies performed for TB.**
    - TB skin test (Mantoux test)

- Chest x-ray
- Bacteriologic studies
- Sputum for AFB Culture

11. What is by tidal volume?

The volume of an inhaled and exhaled air with each breath is called tidal volume. The normal amount is 500ml.

12. What is rhinitis?

Rhinitis is a group of disorders characterized by inflammation and irritation of the mucous membranes of the nose.

13. What is epistaxis?

A hemorrhage from the nose is caused by the rupture of tiny, distended vessels in the mucous membranes of any area of the nose.

14. What is surfactant?

It is a lipoprotein that lowers the surface tension in the alveoli, reduces the amount of pressure needed to inflate the alveoli and decreases the tendency of the alveoli to collapse.

15. Mention the normal breath sounds.

- Vesicular-Soft, low-pitched, gentle, and rustling sounds.
- Bronchovesicular-Medium pitch and intensity
- Bronchial-Louder, high pitched.

16. Mention about abnormal/ adventitious breath sounds.

- Crackles
- Rhonchi
- Wheezes
- Pleural friction rubs.

17. Define thoracentesis.

Thoracentesis is the insertion of a large bore needle through the chest wall into the pleural space to obtain specimens for diagnostic evaluation, remove pleural fluid or instill medication into the pleural space.

18. Define pleural effusion.

Pleural effusion is a collection of fluid in the pleural space.

19. Mention the complications of pulmonary embolism.

- Pulmonary infarction (death of lung tissue).
- Pulmonary hypertension.

20. Mention the management of pulmonary embolism.

- Supplemental oxygen, intubation may be necessary.
- IV for medications and fluid replacement.
- Continuous IV heparin for acute treatments.
- Warfarin for long term therapy.
- Bed rest.
- Opioids for pain relief.
- Pulmonary embolectomy in life threatening situation.

21. What are the indications of chest physiotherapy?

- Excessive bronchial secretions, who has difficulty in clearing secretions with expectorated sputum production greater than 25 ml /day.
- Evidence or suggestion of retained secretions in the presence of an artificial airway.
- Lobar atelectasis caused by or suspected of being caused by mucous plugging.

22. Mention the complications of cystic fibrosis.

- Pneumothorax
- Massive hemoptysis
- Digital clubbing
- Respiratory failure
- Cor pulmonale.

23. Define bronchiectasis.

Bronchiectasis is characterized by permanent abnormal dilatation of one or more large bronchi.

24. Mention the clinical manifestations of bronchiectasis.

- Recurrent cough (sputum 500 ml/day)
- Dyspnea
- Wheezing
- Pleuritic chest pain
- Hemoptysis.

25. List down respiratory and physical therapy for COPD.

- Breathing retraining

Pursed lip breathing

Diaphragmatic breathing

- Effective coughing (huff coughing)
- Chest physiotherapy

Percussion

Vibration

Postural drainage

26. List down the complications of asthma.

- Rib fractures
- Pneumothorax
- Pneumo mediastinum
- Atelectasis
- Pneumonia
- Status asthmaticus.

27. Brief about the pathophysiology of pulmonary hypertension and corpulmonale.

Pulmonary hypertension develops when an occluded vessel impairs the heart's ability to generate enough pressure.This increase in pulmonary vascular resistance progresses to pulmonary hypertension which increases cardiac workload which results in hypertrophy and dilation of right ventricle

28. List down the drug therapy for asthma.

a. Long term medications
- Anti inflammatory drugs

Corticosteroids (inhaled/oral)
- Cromolyn
- Leukotriene modifiers

b. Quick relief medication
- Bronchodilators
- Short acting inhaled ß adrenergic agonists.
- Anti inflammatory drugs
- Corticosteroids.

c. Bronchodilators
- Long acting inhaled ß adrenergic agonists.
- Long acting oral ß adrenergic agonists.
- Theophyline.

29. List out the causes for COPD.

- Cigarette smoking
- Occupational chemicals and dusts.
- Air pollution.
- Respiratory tract infections.
- Hereditary (α1 antitrypsin deficiency)
- Aging (old person)

30. List down the complications of COPD.

- Cor pulmonale.
- Exacerbations of COPD (dyspnea, cough).
- Acute respiratory failure.
- Peptic ulcer and gastroesophageal reflux disease.
- Depression/anxiety.

31. Mention the types of respiratory failure.

Hypoxemic respiratory failure (Type-I)

Hypercapnic respiratory failure (Type-II)

32. Define Fibrothorax.

- It is a complication of emphysema.
- There is fibrous fusion of the visceral and parietal pleura.

33. List out the indications for lung transplantation.

- α 1 antitrypsin deficiency
- Bronchiectasis

- Cystic fibrosis
- Emphysema
- Idiopathic pulmonary fibrosis
- Interstitial lung disease
- Pulmonary hypertension

34. Difference between metered dosed inhaler and dry powder.

Features	Metered dose	Dry powder
Shaking before use	Yes shake well	No
Inspiration	Slow	Rapid
Spacer	Yes at least with inhaled corticosteroids	None permitted
Counting device	No external device	Most preloaded forms
Inhalations/ dose	Often 2/dose	Often 1/dose
Cleaning	Use water for plastic case	Avoid moisture.

35. List down the types of pneumothorax.

- Closed pneumothorax-Accumulation of air in the pleural space.
- Open pneumothorax-Air enters the pleural space through an opening in the chest wall.
- Tension pneumothorax-Rapid accumulation of air in the pleural space.
- Chylthorax-Lymphatic fluid in the pleural space.
- Hemothorax-Accumulation of blood in the interpleural space.

36. List the indications of tracheostomy.

- Bypass an upper airway obstruction.
- Facilitate removal of secretions.
- Permit long term mechanical ventilation.
- Permit oral intake and speech in the patient who requires long term mechanical ventilation.

37. Define pneumonia.

Pneumonia is an acute inflammation of the lung parenchyma caused by a microbial organism like virus, bacteria and fungus.

38. List down the drug therapy for TB.

- Isoniazid
- Rifampicin
- Ethambutol
- Rifabutin
- Pyranamide
- Rifapentine

39. What are fungal infections of the lung?

- Histoplasmosis
- Coccidiodomycosis
- Blastomycosis
- Cryptococcosis
- Aspergillosis
- Candidiasis-Pneumocystitis pneumonia
- Actinomycosis
- Nocardiosis

40. Define Mantoux test.

- The tuberculin skin test is the best way to diagnose latent M. tuberculosis infection.
- Induration at the injection site 48-72 hours after the test means the person has been exposed to TB and has developed antibodies.
- The reaction occurs 2 to 12 weeks after the initial exposure.

41. Define lung abscess.

Lung abscess is a pus containing lesion of the lung parenchyma that gives rise to a cavity. The cavity is formed by necrosis of the lung tissue.

42. List down any four organisms associated with pneumonia.

a) Community acquired pneumonia

- Streptococcus pneumonia
- Mycoplasma pneumonia
- Haemophillus influenzae
- Respiratory viruses
- Chlamydia pneumoniae
- Klebsiella
- Mycobacterium tuberculosis

b) Hospital acquired pneumonia

- Pseudomonas aeruginosa
- Enterobacter
- E.coli
- Proteus
- Klebsiella

43. List the complications of pneumonia.

- Pleurisy
- Pleural effusion
- Atelectasis
- Bactremia
- Lung abscess
- Empyema
- Pericarditis
- Meningitis
- Endocarditis

44. What are indications for pneumococcal vaccine?

- Chronic illnesses such as lung and heart disease and diabetes mellitus.
- Recovering from severe illnesses.
- 65 years of age.
- Long term care.

45. List out clinical manifestations of TB.

- Fatigue
- Malaise
- Anorexia
- Unexplained weight loss
- Low grade fever
- Night sweats.

Test Series III

1. **What is total parenteral nutrition?**
   When the gastrointestinal tract cannot be used for ingestion, digestion and absorption of essential nutrients, TPN may be substituted. TPN is the delivery of a nutritionally adequate hypertonic solution consisting of glucose, protein hydrolysates, minerals and vitamins using an intravenous route.
2. **Define Dumping Syndrome.**
   It occurs with partial gastrectomy; hypertonic, undigested chyme bolus rapidly enters small intestine and pulls fluid into intestine causing decrease in circulating blood volume and increased intestinal peristalsis and motility.
3. **Define ulcerative colitis.**
   Ulcerative colitis is a chronic inflammatory disease of the mucosa and less frequently, the submucosa of the colon and rectum.
4. **Specify the different types of ostomy.**
   - Double barrel colostomy
   - Loop colostomy
   - End colostomy
   - Ileostomy
5. **Classify types of hiatus hernia.**
   - **Sliding hiatal hernia:** Gastroesophageal junction and fundus of stomach slide through the esophageal hiatus.
   - **Paraesophageal hiatal hernia:** The gastroesophageal junction is in normal place but part of stomach herniates through esophageal hiatus; hernia can become strangulated; client may develop gastritis with bleeding.
6. **List down the shunting procedure done for esophageal and gastric varices.**
   - Transjugular Intrahepatic Portosystemic Shunt (TIPS).
   - Portocaval shunt.
   - Distal splenorenal shunt.
7. **Mention common indications for TPN.**
   - Chronic diarrhea and vomiting.
   - Gastrointestinal obstruction.
   - Complicated surgeries or trauma.
   - Malnutrition.
8. **List the causes of appendicitis.**
   - Infection
   - Tumour
   - Fecolith
   - Stricture or intra mural thickening
9. **List complication of ulcerative colitis.**
   - Toxic megacolon
   - Perforation
   - Hemorrhage
   - Malnutrition and anemia

10. Name the complications of hernia.
- GERD
- Esophagitis
- Hemorrhage from erosion
- Stenosis

11. What are the predisposing factors of hernia?
- Increased intra-abdominal pressure
- Increased age
- Trauma
- Congenital weakness
- Forced recumbent position

12. What are the dietary management for irritable bowel syndrome?
- Often benefit from additional dietary fiber: adds bulk and water content to stool, reducing diarrhea and constipation.
- Some benefit from elimination of lactose, fructose and sorbitol.
- Limiting intake of gasforming foods, caffeinated beverages.

13. Mention the purpose of paracentesis.
- Diagnostic purposes.
- To relieve pressure in the organs of the abdomen.
- To instill drugs

14. List down the clinical manifestations of anorexia nervosa.
- Abnormal weight loss.
- Deliberate self starvation.
- Intense fear of gaining weight.
- Lanugo (self, browny hair covering the body except the palms and soles).

15. What is bulimia nervosa?

It is a disorder characterized by frequent binge eating and self induced vomiting associated with loss of control over eating and a persistent concern with body image.

16. Define GERD.

Gastro intestinal esophageal reflux disease is the reflux of gastric contents into the lower esophagus caused by histopathologic alterations.

17. Define Hiatus hernia.

Hiatus hernia is herniation of a portion of the stomach into the esophagus through the opening or hiatus in the diaphragm. It is also referred as diaphragmatic hernia and esophageal hernia.

18. Mention the causes of gastritis.
- Drugs like aspirin. NSAIDS.
- Diet like alcohol, spicy foods.
- Microorganisms like Helicobacter pylori, Salmonella.
- Environmental factors like radiation and smoking.

19. List the causes of peptic ulcer disease.
- Helcobacter pylori
- Burns, NSAIDS
- Stress
- Chronic alcohol consumption and smoking.

20. What is Bilroth I and II surgeries?

Bilroth I – It is partial gastrectomy with removal of the distal two thirds of the stomach and anastomosis of the gastric stump to the duodenum.

Bilroth II-It is partial gastrectomy with removal of the distal two thirds of the stomach and anastomosis of the gastric stump to the jejunum.

21. Mention the postoperative complications of Bilroth I and II surgeries.
- Dumping syndrome
- Postprandial hypoglycemia
- Bile reflux garstritis

22. List triple drug therapy for gastritis.
- Proton pump inhibitor
- Ranitidine bismuth citrate

- Amoxicillin
- Clarithromycin

23. List down the clinical manifestation of peritonitis.

- Abdominal pain
- Rebound tenderness
- Muscular rigidity
- Spasm, paralytic ileus
- Abdominal distention or ascitis

24. Mention the complications of peritonitis.

- Hypovolemic shock
- Septicemia
- Intra abdominal abcess formation
- Paralytic ileus
- Organ failure
- Adhesions or bands

25. Write the stages of appendicitis.

- Simple appendicitis
- Gangrenous appendicitis
- Perforated appendicitis

26. List clinical manifestation of appendicitis.

- Pain in the right lower quadrant.
- Anorexia, nausea and vomiting.
- Rebound tenderness in the Mc Burney's point.
- Constipation or diarrhea.

27. Write any four causes of gastroenteritis. Escherichia coli.

- Staphylococcal food poisoning
- Vibrio cholera
- Salmonella

28. List causes of intestinal obstruction.

- Adhesions
- Strangulated inguinal hernia
- Illeocecal intussuseption
- Volvulus
- Mesenteric occlusion
- Neoplasm

29. What are the types of stomatitis?

- Aphthous stomatitis
- Nicotine stomatitis
- Herpetic gingivostomatitis

30. Mention the causes of oral cancer.

- Over exposure to sun
- Ruddy and fair complexion
- Recurrent herpetic lesion
- Tobacco use
- Poor oral hygiene
- Chronic alcohol intake

31. Define Leukoplakia and erythroplakia.

- Leukoplakia – The white patch or smoker's patch is often a precancerous lesion in mucous of mouth/tongue.
- Erythroplakia – Red velvety patch on the mouth or tongue.

32. List down the surgeries for oral cance.

- Partial madibulectomy.
- Hemiglossectomy
- Glossectomy
- Resection of buccal mucosa and floor of mouth
- Radical neck dissection

33. Brief about xerostomia.

It is the dryness of mouth when exposed to radiation and among mouth breathers.

Treatment – Use of humidifier, use of synthetic saliva, intake of adequate fluids. Avoid dry bulky and irritating food.

34. What are surgeries for ulcerative colitis?

- Total proctocolectomy with permanent ileostomy.
- Total proctocolectomy with continent ileostomy.
- Total colectomy with rectal mucosal strip.
- Total proctocolectomy with ileal reservoir.

35. What are the types of upper GI bleeding?

- Hematemesis

- Malena
- Occult blood

36. Define ostomy.

An ostomy is the surgical procedure in which an opening is made to allow the passage of intestinal contents from the bowel to to an incision or stoma.

37. What are the types of hernia?

- Hiatus hernia
- Inguinal hernia
- Umbilical hernia
- Incisional hernia
- Femoral hernia

38. Write the four differences between gastric ulcer and duodenal ulcer.

S. no	Character-istics	Gastric ulcer	Duodenal ulcer
1	Lesion	superficial	Penetrating
2	Location	Antrum, body and fundus	Duodenum
3	Gastric secretion	Normal to decreased	increased
4	Incidence	Greater in women	Greater in men

39. Name the four types of cirrhosis of liver.

- Alcoholic cirrhosis
- Post necrotic cirrhosis
- Biliary cirrhosis
- Cardiaç cirrhosis

40. List complications of cirrhosis of liver.

- Portal hypertension
- Hepatic encephalopathy
- Esophageal varices
- Ascitis

41. What are complications of hepatitis?

- Fulminant hepatitis
- Chronic hepatitis
- Cirrhosis of liver
- Hepatocellular carcinoma

42. Define Gastroesophageal Reflux Disease.

Gastroesophageal reflux is the backward flow of gastric content into the esophagus.

43. What are the factors contributing to gastroesophageal reflux?

- Increased gastric volume (post meals)
- Position pushing gastric contents close to gastro esophageal juncture (such as bending or lying down).
- Increased gastric pressure (obesity or tight clothing.
- Hiatal hernia.

44. Define achalasia.

It is characterized by impaired peristalsis of smooth muscle of esophagus and impaired relaxation of lower esophageal sphincter.

45. What are complications of radiation therapy?

Perforation, hemorrhage, stricture

46. List down treatment of peptic ulcer.

Rest and stress reduction

Nutritional management

Pharmacological management

Antacids (Mylanta)-Neutralizes acids

Proton pump inhibitors (Prilosec, Prevacid)-Blocks gastric acid secretion.

47. Mention the surgical intervention for peptic ulcer.

- Minimally invasive gastrectomy.
- Partial gastric removal with laproscopic surgery.
- Bilroth I and II.
- Removal of portions of the stomach.
- Vagotomy.
- Cutting of the vagus nerve to decrease

acid secretion.

- Pyloroplasty.
- Widens the pyloric sphincter.

48. What are the causes of peritonitis?

- Ruptured appendix
- Perforated bowel secondary to PUD
- Diverticulitis
- Gangrenous gall bladder
- Ulcerative colitis
- Trauma
- Peritoneal dialysis

49. What are complications of peritonitis?

- Abscess
- Fibrous adhesions
- Septicemia, septic shock, fluid loss into abdominal cavity leads to hypovolemic shock.

50. What is the treatment for peritonitis?

- Broadspectrum antibiotics before definitive culture results identifying specific organism(s) causing infection is identified.
- Analgesics.
- Laparotomy to treat cause (close perforation, remove inflammed tissue).
- Peritoneal Lavage: washing out peritoneal cavity with copious amounts of warm isotonic fluid during surgery to dilute residual bacterial and remove gross contaminants.

51. What is continent (or Kock's) ileostomy?

Continent (or Kock's) ileostomy has intra-abdominal reservoir with nipple valve formation to allow catheter insertion to drain out stool.

52. What are complications of ulcerative colitis?

- Hemorrhage toxic megacolon.
- Increased risk for colorectal cancer.
- Abcess, fistula formation.
- Bowel obstruction.

53. What is toxic megacolon?

It usually involves transverse colon which dilates and lacks peristalsis leads to colon perforation.

Manifestations: fever, tachycardia, hypotension, dehydration, change in stools, abdominal cramping.

54. List medications for ulcerative colitis.

- **Sulfasalazine (Azulfidine):** Salicylate compound that inhibits prostaglandin production to reduce inflammation.
- **Corticosteroids:** Reduce inflammation and induce remission; with ulcerative colitis may be given as enema; intravenous steroids are given with severe exacerbations.
- Immunosuppressive agents (azathioprine (Imuran), cyclosporine) for clients who do not respond to steroid therapy alone.

55. What are complications of peptic ulcer?

- Hematemesis
- Melena
- Hematochezia (blood in stool)
- Gastric outlet (pyloric sphincter) obstruction
- Anemia

56. List manifestations of gastric cancer.

Early satiety, anorexia, indigestion, vomiting, pain after meals not responding to antacids, weight loss, cachexia (wasted away appearance), abdominal mass, stool positive for occult blood.

57. Define dumping syndrome.

Occurs with partial gastrectomy; hypertonic, undigested chyme bolus rapidly enters small intestine and pulls fluid into intestine causing decrease in circulating blood volume and increased intestinal peristalsis and motility.

58. Define post prondial hypoglycaemia.

Post prondial hypoglycaemia occurs 2-3 hours after meal. Symptoms of hypoglycemia in response to excessive release of insulin that occurred from rise in blood glucose when chyme entered intestine.

59. Mention contraindication of liver biopsy.

- Bleeding disorder.
- Infections – such as liver abcess, hydatid cyst.
- Severe hepatocellular jaundice.
- Gross ascitis.
- Haemangioma of liver.

60. Mention complications of liver biopsy.

- Hemorrhage.
- Hypovolemic shock

61. What are causes of liver abcess?

- Entamoeba histolytica
- Poor sanitation
- Poor hygiene

62. What is paracentesis?

Paracentesis the removal of fluid (ascitis) from the peritoneal cavity through a small surgical incision or puncture made through the abdominal wall under sterile conditions.

63. What are the types of jaundice?

- Hemolytic jaundice
- Hepatocellular jaundice
- Obstructive jaundice

64. Write down the clinical manifestation of peritonitis.

- Abdominal pain
- Rebound tenderness
- Muscular rigidity
- Spasm, paralytic ileus
- Abdominal distention or ascites

65. Define fulminant hepatic failure.

Fulminant hepatic failure is the clinical syndrome of sudden and severely impaired liver function in a previously healthy person.

66. Difference between ulcerative colitis and crohn's disease.

S. no	charecter-istics	Ulcerative colitis	Chrohn's disease
1	Location	Start in the rectum or sigmoid colon	Occur anywhere along the GI tract
2	Distribution	Spreads in a continuous pattern	Occurs as skip lesion
3	Depth of involvement	Mucosa and submucosa	Entire thickness of bowel wall
4	Granulomas	Absent	Common

67. How to assess the abdominal wave or fluid thrill ?

The examiner places the hands along the side of the patient's flank, then strikes one flank sharply, detecting any fluid wave with the other hand. An assistants's hand is placed along the patient midline to prevent the fluid wave from being transmitted through the tissues of the abdominal wall.

68. What are the types of jaundice?

- Hemolytic jaundice
- Hepatocellular jaundice
- Obstructive jaundice

69. Mention the risk factors for the transmission of hepatitis B.

- Frequent exposure to infected blood and blood products.
- Sexual activity with the infected person.

Test Series IV

1. **Define anemia.**
   Anemia is defined as a reduction in the concentration of hemoglobin in the peripheral blood below the normal for the age and sex of the patient.
2. **Write down the classifications of anemia.**
   1. **Acquired anemia**
      - Iron deficiency anemia
      - Pernicious anemia
      - Aplastic anemia
      - Anemia due to bone marrow failure
      - Anemia caused by folic acid deficiency
   2. **Hemolytic anemia**
      - Hemolysis caused by trauma
      - Hemolysis caused by infectious agents
   3. **Hemorrhagic anemia**
      - Acute hemorrhagic anemia
      - Chronic hemorrhagic anemia
   4. **Congenital anemias**
      - Sickle cell anemia
      - Thalassemia
3. **List clinical manifestation of anemia.**
   - Dyspnea
   - Palpitations
   - Diaphoresis
   - Chronic fatigue
   - Pallor – pallor of the nail buds, mucous membranes of the mouth and conjunctivae.
   - Numbness
   - Amenorrhoea & menorrhagia in female
   - Loss of libido in males
   - Lack of concentration
   - Tingling of hands and feet.
   - Bone pain
   - Anorexia
   - Headache, vertigo
   - Hepatomegaly, spleenomegaly
4. **List out the causes of anemia.**
   - Excessive blood loss.
   - Deficiencies and abnormalities of red blood cell production.
   - Excessive destruction of red blood cells.
   - Poor nutrition.
5. **What are the acquired causes of anemia?**
   - Iron deficiency anemia
   - Pernicious anemia
   - Aplastic anemia
   - Anemia due to bone marrow failure
   - Anemia caused by folic acid deficiency.
6. **Write about the therapeutic management of anemia.**
   - Supportive care – Bedrest, oxygen administrator

- Antibiotic
- Analgesic for pain
- Iron supplement
- Transfusion therapy
- Hydroxyurea therapy – increases Hb
- levels and reduces hemolysis.

7. What are the characteristics of hemolytic anemia?

Hemolytic anemia is a condition in which red blood cells are destroyed and removed from the bloodstream. Characteristics include normocytic, normochromic anemia.

- Shortened RBC survival.
- Reticulocytosis-response to increased RBC destruction.
- Increased indirect bilirubin.
- Increased LDH.

8. What are findings of hemolytic anemia?

- Less hemoglobin count
- Hemoglobinuria
- Hemoglobinemia

9. What are the causes of hemolytic anemia?

Intracorpuscular Hemolysis

Membrane Abnormalities
Metabolic Abnormalities
Hemoglobinopathies

Extracorpuscular Hemolysis

Nonimmune
Immune

Hemolytic anemia is caused by

- Hemolysis caused by trauma
- Hemolysis caused by infectious agents
- Hemolysis caused by systemic disease

10. What are the membrane defects leading to hemolytic anemia?

- **Microskeletal defects**

Hereditary spherocytosis

- **Membrane permeability defects**

Hereditary stomatocytosis

- **Increased sensitivity to complement**

Paroxysmal nocturnal hemoglobinuria

11. What is pernicious anemia?

Pernicious anemia is a type of anemia due to failure of absorption of vitamin B12.

12. Mention the major characteristics of pernicious anemia.

- Abnormally large red blood cells
- Hypochlorhydria
- Neurologic and gastro intestinal manifestation
- A fatal outcome unless the client receives life long injections of vitamin B12

13. Write the etiology and risk factors for pernicious anemia.

- Lack of intrinsic factor due to atrophy of the stomach glandular mucosa.
- Heredity.
- Prolonged iron deficiency anemia.
- Gastric resection.

14. Write about the clinical features of pernicious anemia.

- Sore tongue
- Anorexia
- Nausea
- Vomiting
- Abdominal pain
- Weakness and paresthesias of the feet and hand
- Reduced vibratory and position senses
- Ataxia
- Muscle weakness

15. List out the clinical manifestation of sickle cell anemia.

- Bone pain
- Chest pain
- Cardiomegaly
- Chronic fatigue
- Jaundice
- Joint swelling

- Pallor
- Tachycardia
- Hepatomegaly
- Increased susceptibility to infection

16. What is thrombocytopenia?

Thrombocytopenia is a reduction of platelets below the normal range of 150,000 to 400,000/ml (150-400 x 109/L).

17. What is lymphoma?

Lymphomas are malignant neoplasms originating in the bone marrow and lymphatic structures resulting in the proliferation of lymphocytes.

18. Mention the types of lymphoma.

- Hodgkin's disease
- Non-Hodgkin's Lymphoma

19. Define Hodgkin's lymphoma.

Neoplastic disorder with development of specific infiltrate containing pathologic Reed-Sternberg cells. It usually arises in lymph nodes and spreads to contigeuous groups. Extranodal presentation is rare. Disease is associated with defective cellular immunity.

20. Mention three major disorders of hemostasis.

- Thrombocytopenia.
- Hemophilia and Von Willebrand disease.
- Disseminated intravascular coagulation.

21. List common disorders of the veins.

- Venous thrombosis
- Thrombophelebitis
- Deep vein thrombosis

22. What is iron deficiency anemia and what are its causes?

It is defined as anemia associated with either inadequate absorption or excessive loss of iron; it is a chronic, microcytic, hypochromic anemia.

Causes are:

- Inadequate dietary intake
- Mal absorption
- Blood loss or hemolysis
- Pregnancy
- Chronic renal failure
- Dialysis

23. Mention the diagnostic studies for iron deficiency anemias.

- History & physical examination
- HCT and HB levels
- Reticulocyte count
- Serum iron
- Serum ferritin
- Stool for occult blood

24. Write the therapeutic management for iron deficiency anemia.

- Identification and treatment of underlying cause
- Administration of ferrous sulfate or ferrous gluconate
- Administration of iron dextron IM or IV
- Diet rich in foods containing iron
- Nutritional education
- Transfusion of packed RBCs

25. Write the clinical features of iron deficiency anemia.

- Pallor
- Glossitis
- Cheilitis
- Palpitation
- Dizziness
- Sensitivity to cold
- Headache
- Burning sensation of the tongue
- Elevated leukocyte and uric acid, vitamin B12 levels

26. What is bone marrow?

Bone marrow is the soft material that fills

the central core of bones. It is the blood-forming tissue that produces the three major cell components of the blood: Red (Erythrocytes) blood cells (RBC's), White (Leukocytes) blood cells (WBCs) and platelets.

27. What are common causes of folic acid deficiency?

- Poor nutrition
- Mal absorption syndromes
- Drugs – methotrexate, oral contraceptives and anticonvulsants
- Alcohol abuse and anorexia

28. List out clinical manifestation of acute blood loss.

- Tachy cardia
- Hypotension
- Decreased CVP
- Decreased cardiac out put
- Cold and clammy extremities
- Shock and potential death

29. Mention the etiology of an aplastic anemia.

- Congenital
- **Acquired** – Exposure to ionizing radiation, chemical agents, viral and bacterial infection (hepatitis, military TB) and medications.

30. Write about therapeutic management for aplastic anemia.

- Replacing blood volume to prevent stock
- Identifying the source of the hemorrhage and stop the blood loss.
- I.V. fluids (Dextron, Hetastrach, albumin).

31. What is sickle cell anemia?

It is a congenital hemolytic anemia. It results from a defective Hb molecule, which causes RBCs to roughness and become sickle shaped and more fragile.

32. Mention etiology of sickle cell anemia.

It is an autosomal recessive genetic disorder in which the person is homozygous for Hbs.

33. Write about symptoms of sickle cell crisis.

Severe abdominal, thoracic, muscular or bone pain

- Low grade fever
- Increased jaundice and dark urine
- Difficulty awakening
- Irritability
- Lethargy & Listlessness
- Blood – Hb & RBCs
- Serum bilirubin
- Skeletal X rays to see the bone & joint deformities
- MRI to see the blockage of cerebral vessels

34. What is polycythemia?

Polycythemia is the production and presence of increased numbers of RBCs.

35. Mention the types of polycythemia.

- Primary polycythemia or polycythemia vera
- Secondary polycythemia

36. Write the clinical manifestations of polycythemia.

- Headache • Vertigo • Dizziness
- Tinnitus • Visual disturbances
- Angina • Thrombophlebitis

37. Mention the complication of polycythemia.

- G.I. bleeding or epistaxis
- Hepatomegaly
- Splenomegaly.
- Plethora
- Hyper uricemia

38. Write about diagnostic studies.

- Elevated Hb and RBC count
- Elevated WBC with basophils
- Elevated platelets

- Supportive care – Bedrest, oxygen administrator
- Antibiotic
- Analgesic for pain
- Iron supplement
- Transfusion therapy
- Hydroxyurea therapy – increases Hb levels and reduces hemolysis.

39. What is polycythemia vera?

Polycythemia vera is classified as a myloproliferative disorder (meaning over growth of bone marrow).

40. What is hemophilia?

It is a hereditary bleeding disorder, caused by defective or deficient coagulation factors.

41. What is thrombotic thrombocytopenia purpura?

It is an uncommon syndrome characterized by microangiopathic, hemolytic anemia, thrombocytopenia, neurologic abnormalities, fever and renal abnormalities.

42. What is disseminated intravascular coagulation?

DIC is a serious bleeding disorder resulting from abnormally initiated and accelerated clotting.

43. What is leukemia?

It is a group of malignant disorders affecting the blood and blood-forming tissues of the bone marrow, lymphsystem and spleen.

44. Mention the types of leukemia.

- Acute myelogenous leukemia.
- Acute lymphocytic leukemia.
- Chronic myelogenous leukemia.
- Chronic lymphocytic leukemia.

45. Write about the etiology and risk factors of leukemia.

- Genetic and environmental factors
- Chemical agents (eg) benzene
- Chemotherapeutic agents (eg) alkylating agent
- Viruses
- Radiation exposure

46. List out the clinical manifestation of Leukemia.

Fatigue & weakness.

- Headache
- Fever
- Pallor, bleeding
- Anorexia
- Anemia
- Mouth sore
- Joint pain
- Hepatosplenomegaly
- Lymphadenopathy
- CNS involvement

47. Write about the chemotherapeutic agents used to treat leukemia.

- Alkylating agents – Cyclophorsphamide
- Antitumor antibiotics – Doxorubicin
- Anti metabolities – Methotrexate
- Corticosteriod – Prednisone
- Nitroso ureas – Carmustine
- Plant alkaloid – Vincristine
- Miscellaneous – L. aspargienase

48. Mention the types of hemophilias.

Hemophilia A (Classic hemophilia)

- Hemophilia B (Christmas disease)
- Von Willebrand's disease

Test Series V

1. **What is Raynaud's phenomenon?**
   Raynaud's phenomenon is an episodic vasospastic disorder of small cutaneous arteries, most frequently involving the fingers and toes.
2. **What is hypertension?**
   Hypertension or high Blood pressure is defined as persistent elevation of systolic blood pressure > 140 mm Hg, Diastolic blood pressure > 90 mm of Hg, or using Antihypertensive medication.
3. **What are the non modifiable risk factors for primary hypertension?**
   Family History: Close blood relative like parents or siblings.
   Obesity: Weight gain after 18 years of more than 5 kg especially central abdominal obesity.
   Ethnicity: High in Africans and Asians.
   Sedentary: Physical activity.
   Social economic status: Hypertension is more in lower socio economic group and among less educated.
   Stress: Person exposed to repeated stress and responding differently to stress. Physiological response to stress in ↑ d SNS activity.
4. **What is a hypertensive crisis?**
   Severe abrupt elevation in BP arbitrarily define as a DBP >14 mm Hg.
5. **What are the causes of hypertensive crisis?**
   Exacerbation of chronic HT, Renovascular HT, Preeclampsia, eclampsia, pheochromocytoma, Drugs Acetaminophine, MOI, Rebound HT.
6. **What is the collaborative management of CAD?**
   Nutritional Therapy: 30% of total calories from fat mainly mono unsaturated fats in nuts and oils, complex carbohydrates with whole grains, fruits, and omega-3 fatty acids, EPA and DHA from fatty fish such as salmon and tuna. Controlling weight and avoidance of tobacco and using cholesterol lowering drugs.
7. **What are the major treatment elements of chronic stable angina?**
   - ACE Inhibitors
   - β-Adrenergic blockers to control Bloodpressure
   - Avoiding cigarette smoking: For cholestrol
   - Dietcontrol: For diabeties patients
   - Education: Exercise

8. What are the investigations done for aneurysms?

- Chest X Ray, PFT
- ECG, Echo
- ESR
- Urea & Electrolytes
- USD (DOPPLER)
- Spiral CT with contrast
- Arteriography

9. What are the cellular changes in heart failure?

Changes in Ca^{+2} handling.
Changes in adrenergic receptors:
Slight ↑ in α1 receptors
β_1 receptors desensitization → followed by down regulation
Changes in contractile proteins
Program cell death (Apoptosis)
Increase amount of fibrous tissue

10. What are the diagnostic tests done for rheumatic heart disease?

- RA Factor
- WBC and ESR
- C-reactive protein
- Cardiac enzymes
- EKG
- Chest x-ray
- Echo
- Cardiac catheterization
- Cardiac output

11. What is the nursing management for valvular disorders?

- O2 as prescribed
- Emotional support, patient and family education
- Administer medications
- Intake output chart weight
- Check for edema

12. What are clinical manifestations of hypertensive crisis?

Sudden rise in BP associated with headache, nausea, vomiting, seizures, confusion, stupor and coma due to increased capillary permeability leading to cerebral edema. Blurred vision and transient blindness from papilledema and retinopathy, renal insufficiency can also occur.

13. What are the cholesterol lowering drugs?

I. Drugs that restrict lipoprotein production:

- STATIN group of drugs such as lovastatin, atorvastatin which inhibit synthesis of cholesterol by blocking HMG-COA reductase.
- NIACIN – A water soluable vitamin lowers LDL & triglyceride
- FIBRIC ACID DERIVATIVES- Accelerate elimination of VLDL effective in lowering tryglycerides such as Fenofibrate.

II Drugs that increase lipoprotien removal bile acid sequestrants by conversions of cholesterol to bile acids such as cholestyramine.

III Drugs that decrease cholesterol absorption:

Ezetimibe inhibits absorption of dietary and biliary cholesterol

IV Antiplatelet therapy:

Aspirin and clopidrogel for patients with a risk of ≥10%

14. What is angina?

Angina is chest pain caused due to reversible myocardial ischemia when there is an increased demand for oxygen or decreased supply of myocardial oxygen by the coronary arteries.

15. What are the types of angina?

Chronic Stable Angina: Chest pain that occurs intermittently over a long period with same pattern of onset, duration and intensity of symptoms.

Silent Ischemia: Refers to ischemia that occurs in the absence of subjective symptoms seen in diabetic patients due to autonomic neuropathy.

Nocturnal Angina: Occurs only at night, but not necessarily while lying down.

Prinzmetal's Angina (Variant Angina): Occurs in response to a spasm of coronary artery stimulated by factors such as the myocardial O2 demand in absence of CAD or physical demand and increased levels of certain substances such as histamine, angiotensin, epinephrine, norepinephrine and prostaglandin.

16. What are the contra indications of IABP?

- Irreversible brain damage
- Terminal or untreatable disease of any major organ system
- Abdominal aortic and thoracic aneurysm
- Moderate to severe aortic insufficiency
- Generalized peripheral vascular disease

17. What are the mechanical circulatory assist devices?

- IABP
- Left or right ventricular assistive devices (VAD)
- VAD's provide in turn support in three types if situation.
- Left, right or both ventricles support while recovering from acute injury.
- Heart requires surgical repair but patient must be stabilized.
- Heart has failed and the patient is awaiting cardiac transplantation.

18. What are the complications of mechanical ventilation?

- Ventilator associated pneumonia
- Baro trauma
- Bronchospasm
- Muscle damage
- Pulmonary bleeding

19. What are the mechanisms regulating blood pressure?

Blood Pressure is regulated by complex short term mechanisms such as the SNS and vascular endothelium within a few seconds. Long term mechanisms include renal and hormonal processes that regulate arteriolar resistance and blood volume.

20. What are the clinical manifestations of hypertension?

Asymptomtic symptoms due to effects on blood vessels in various organs or increased workload to the heart.

Secondary symptoms include fatigue, reduced activity tolerance, dizzyness, palpitations, angina and dyspnea, IV High BP, headache, nose bleed and dizziness.

21. What are the drugs used in the management of CSA?

Short acting nitrates: Which dilates peripheral blood vessels and coronary arteries and collateral vessels-IV, subsequently or transligually, transdermal patch.

Anti platelets agents: Asprin that inhibits cyclooxygenase and reducing the platelet activator, thrombose A2 and adenesine diphospate receptor antagonist like clopidogrel.

β adrenergic blockers: Atenolol to heart rate.

22. What are the symptoms of heart failure?

- SOB, orthopnea, paroxysmal nocturnal dyspnea
- Low cardiac output symptoms
- Abdominal symptoms: Anorexia, nausea, abdominal fullness, right hypochondrial pain.

23. What are the pathophysiological changes in mitral stenosis?

- Rheumatic carditis is a thickening by fibrosis or calcification by tumors, calcium and thrombus.
- Valve leaflets fuse and become stiff and the cordae tendinea contract.
- These narrow the opening and prevents normal blood flow from the LA to the LV, LA pressure increases, left atrium dilates, PAP increases, and the RV hypertrophies, Pulmonary congestion and right sided heart failure occurs, Followed by decreased preload and CO decreases.

24. What is surgical management for valvular disorders?

- Mitral Valve
- Commissurotomy
- Mitral Valve Replacement
- Balloon Valvuloplasty
- Aortic Valve Replacement with biological (tissue), porcine valve and Mechanical valve

25. What are the types of shock?

- Cardiogenic shock
- Hypovolemic shock
- Neurogenic shock
- Anaphylactic shock
- Septic shock

26 What are the drugs used for hypertensive emergencies?

Vasodilators such as sodium nitroprusside, NTG, feroldopam, hydralazine, nicardipine adrenergic blocking agents such as phentolamine, labetalol, esmolol and ACE inhibitors such as enalapril are used.

27 How to measure CVP?

Using one of the proximal lumen or with central venous catheter in the internal jugular or subclavian vein.

28. List the relative contra indication of VAD.

- BSA less than 1.5 m2
- Renal or liver failure.
- Comorbidities that could limit life expectancy to lesst than 3 years.

29. What are disadvantages of nasal ET.

- Kinking/ narrowing tube
- Suction the secretion difficult

30. What are the indications of IABP?

- Refractory unstable angina
- Short term bridge of cardiac transplant
- High risk interventional cardiology procedures
- Pre, intra and postoperative cardiac surgery

31. What is SIMV mode of ventilation?

Rate, VT, inspiratory time sensitivity &PEEP are set by doctor in between the mandatory breaths it can breathe spontaneously, breath at the own rates with preset Fio2.

32. What is the role of the SNS in regulating BP?

The baroreceptors (presso receptors) located in the carotid artery and the arch of aorta sense changes in (stretching) BP and transmit it to the vasomotor centres in the medulla of brainstem. This information is relayed throughout the brain by the network of exciting or inhibiting efferent nerves, innervating the cardiac and vascular smooth muscles. Norepinephrine, the neurotransmitter released from the SNS nerve endings, activates the receptors located in the SA node, myocardium, increases the heart rate and cardiac contractility & speed of conduction and vascular smooth muscle, which causes vasoconstriction in the peripheral arterioles thereby the cardiac output.

Release of renin from the kidneys leading to increased arterial pressure.

33. How do kidneys regulate blood pressure?

The kidneys control the excretion of sodium and lead to retention of water causing increased ECF volume and increased venous return to the heart and elevated BP by increasing cardiac output.

34. What is the role of the renin angiotensin aldosterone system in BP regulation?

Renin is secreted from the juxtaglomerular apparatus in the kidney in response to SNS stimulation, decreased blood flow through the kidneys or decreased sodium concentration. The enzyme rennin converts angiotensinogen to angiotensin-I. Angiotensin converting enzyme (ACE) converts angiotensin I into angiotensin II, a potent vasoconstrictor and an immediate increase in BP. Also over a period of hours or days angiotensin II stimulates the adrenal cortex to secrete aldosterone which causes sodium and water retention. This process is also called the renin-angiotensin–aldosterone system.

35. Describe classification of hypertension.

Blood pressure of <120 /80 mm of Hg is normal. Prehypertension is SBP 120-139 or DBP 80-89.

36. What are the subtypes of hypertension?

Isolated systolic hypertension is defined as an average SBP ≥ 140 mmhg coupled with DBP <90mm hg and is comman in older adult due to loss of elasticity from other arteriosclerosis.

Pseudo hypertension (also Hypertension) can occur with advanced calcified asteriosclerosis in which sclerotic arteries do not collapse even when cuff is fully inflated. The only way to accurately measure BP is through inter areterial catheter.

37. What is secondary hypertension?

Secondary HT is elevated BP with a specific identifiable causes of secondary hypertension are coarctation or congenital narrowing of aorta, renal disease like renal artery stenosis and parenchymal disease, endocrine disorders such as phechromocytoma, cushing's disease and hyperaldosteronisum. Neurological disorder such as brain tumors, tetraplegia and head injury, sleep apnea, medications such as sympathetic stimulants, oral contraceptive, NSAID, cirhosis & pregnancy induced hypertension.

38. What are the risk factors for primary hypertension?

Age: After 50 an SBP > 140 mm Hg

Alcohol: Excessive alcohol intake > 1 ounce of alcohol, smoking.

DM: When HT coexists largest organ disease is more common due to insulin resistance and hyperinsulinemia.

Gender: Men in adulthood and early middle age < 55 years of age and in Women >55 years of age.

39. What is acute coronary syndrome?

Unstable angina and myocardial infarction are the more serious manifestations of CAD and are termed as acute coronary Syndrome (ACS)

40. What is coronary artery disease?

It is a type of blood vessel disorder involving coronary arteries due to atherosclerosis, the hardening of fatty bunch in arteries.

41. What is etiology of CAD?

Arteriosclerosis is the major cause of CAD characterized by focal deposit of cholesterol and lipids (atheromas) with in the internal wall of arteries.

The endothelial lining can be injured due to tobacco, hyperlipidemia and hypertension. Elevation of C-reactive protein, a non specific marker can lead to rupture of plaque and oxidation of LDL cholesterol.

42. List the aspects of primary survey.

- Airway with cervical spine stabilisation and immobilisation
- Breathing
- Circulation
- Disability

43. List the causes of life threatening conditions identified during primary survey.

Airway : Inhalation injury, obstruction, penetrating or blunt trauma to upper airway structure.

Breathing : Anaphylaxis, flail chest with pulmonary contusion, pneumothorax, hemothorax.

Circulation : Direct cardiac injury, pericardial tamponade, shock, uncontrolled external haemorrhage.

Disability : Head injury, stroke.

44. Mention the signs of successful CPR.

- Normal heart rate
- Restoration of BP
- Normal respiratory rate
- Normal ECG

45. Mention diagnostic test for brain death.

Coma, unresponsiveness, absence of brain reflexes, apnea.

46. What are the common complications of hypertension?

- The common complications of hypertension are target organ diseases occurring in the heart (hypertensive heart) disease,
- Brain (cerebro vascular disease)
- Peripheral vascular disease,
- Kidney (nephro sclerosis) and
- Eye (retinal damage).

47. What are the diagnostic studies in hypertension?

H/E, P/ E, ECG, Total lipid, Triglyceride, Echo Glucose, HDL, LFT, Serium Na, K, Cl, Co2, Ca, LDL, TSH, BUN creatinine. Total to HDL ratio, CBC, Uric acid.

48. What are collaborative therapies for hypertension?

- Nutritional Therapy: In take of pottassium, fruits and vegetables, ↓<6gm/day or 2.4 gm of sodium salt and restrict cholesteral and saturated fats. Low fat dairy products for calcium and magnesium, lot of water.
- Regulate, moderate physical activity-30mts/day. Brisk walking, jogging, swimming→ to ↓ SBP to 9mm Hg
- Weight control 10 kg weight loss→↓SBP of 5 to 20 mm Hg
- Moderation of alcohol to <1.5 ounce /day
- Avoidance of tobacco
- Stress Management: By relaxation therapy, guided imagery and Biofeedback.

49. What are the drugs used in the treatement of hypertension?

Thiazide Diverties → benzechlor trichlormenthhydrothiazde.

Loop Diuretics → bumentide, Furosemide.

Potassium sparing Diuretics → amiloride, Triamterene

Aldosterone receptor blocker → Sprionolactone, eplereone

Adrenergic inhibitors → guanfacine, methyldopa

50. What are developmental stages in CAD?

The stages of development of Arteriosclerosis are fatty streak, fibrous plaque due to smooth muscle cell proliferation and complicated lesion.

51. What is fatty streak?

Fatty streak is the earliest lesion of arteriosclerosis and characterized by lipid filled smooth muscle cells leading to fatty streaks with yellow fringe.

52. What is fibrous plaque?

Fibrous plaque is the progressive changes in endothelium of arterial wall in a patient with CAD where endothelial injury causes LDL growth.

Factors from platelets stimulate smooth muscle proliferation and thickening of arterial wall. Lipoprotiens transport cholesterol and other lipids to the arterial intima. The fatty streak is covered by collanger formula fibrous plaque appears grayish or wheatish. Plaques can form on one portion of artery or in a circular fashion occluding the lumen.

53. What is complicated lesion?

The fibrous plaque grows continued inflammation can result in plaques, instability, ulceration and rupture.

Platelets can accumulate in large numbers leading to a thrombus and cause further narrowing or total occlusion of the artery.

54. Which are the artificial airways used?

- Endotracheal intubation
- Oral
- Nasal
- Tracheostomy

55. What are the indications for endotracheal intubation?

- Upper airway obstruction
- Trauma
- Respiratory distress
- Decreased

56. What are advantages of oral intubation?

- Minimal nostril injury
- Easy to intubate

57. What are disadvantages of oral intubation.

- It may be difficult to place on oral tube, its head & neck mobility is limited.
- Teeth can be clipped or dislodged during the procedure.

58. Mention the advantages of Nasal ET.

- More stable than oral tube
- Mouth care to be accompanied

59. Brief about the interpretation for CVP.

- **Increased CVP** Right ventricular failure or volume overload
- **Decreased CVP** Hypovolemia.

60. What are the factors causing decreased myocardial oxygen supply?

Decreased oxygen supply is through the non cardiac factors of anemia, hyper mania, pneumonia, asthma, COPD and hypovolemia, cardiac factors such as coronary artery spasm, coronary artery thrombosis, dysrthythmias, heart failure, valve disorders.

61. What are the factors leading to increased oxygen demand or consumption?

The non cardiac factors are anxiety, cocaine use, hypertension, hypothermia, hyperthyroidism and physical exertion. The cardiac factors are physical exertion, aortic stenosis, cardiomyopathy, dysrhythamias, tachycardias.

62. Describe PQRST assessment of angina.

Assess: Precipitating factors such as exercise, rest

Ask: The quality of pain such as dull, acute, tight, squeezing, enquire radiation of pain to back, arms, jaw, teeth, shoulder and elbow.

Severity of pain could be graded on a scale

of 0 to 10.

Timing of when the pain began, previous pain and change in the pain overtime should be found

63. What are the precipitating factors of angina?

- Physical exertion
- Temperature extremes
- Strong emotion
- Consumption of a heavy meal
- Nicotine in Tobacco

64. Describe pain in CSA.

Most of the pain appears subsequently with pain radiating to jaw, shoulder, and down the arm. The other various locations are upper chest; epigastric, left shoulder and intra scapular.

The pain may be constrictive, squeezing, heavy, choking or suffocating sensation or just complaints of indigestion or burning sensation in epigastric region.

65. Define aneurysms.

Permanent localized dilatation of the affected artery over the normal diameter

- 50% Arteriomegaly
- 100% Aneurysms

As the age increases, arteries become stiffer, wider (aneurysm) and longer (tortousity).

66. What is the etiology of aneurysms?

- Most aneurysms are caused by degenerative disease affecting the vessel (atherosclerosis)
- Structural weakness & Haemodynamic forces
  - Damage to intimal hyperplasia
  - Reduction in the elastin and collagen content of the media
  - Collagen; tensile strength, adventitia
  - Elastin; recoil capacity, media
- Risk factors
  - smoking, hypertension, hypercholesterolaemia

67. What is management for aneurysms?

- Elective repair for AAA >6cm
- Mortality 5%
- Urgent repair for AAA <6cm
- Developed back pain
- Rate of growth >0.5cm/6 month
- Emergency repair for ruptured AAA
- Mortality 50%

68. What are the rare causes of aneurysms?

- Congenital
- Marfan's syndrome, Berry aneurysms
- Post-stenotic
- Coarctation of the aorta, cervical rib, popliteal artery entrapment syndrome
- Traumatic
- Gunshot, stab wounds, arterial punctures
- Inflammatory
- Takayasu's disease, Behcet's disease, Mycotic
- Bacterial endocarditis, syphilis
- Pregnancy associated
- Splenic, cerebral, aortic, renal, iliac & coronary

69. Describe the classification of aneurysms.

False

Due to traumatic breach in the wall

The sac made up from the compressed surrounding tissue

True

Dilatation involving all layers of the wall

Fusiform

Spindle-shaped involving whole circumference

Saccular

Small segment of wall ballooning due to localized weakness

Depending on location

Abdominal aortic aneurysms
Femoral
Popiliteal
Spleenic

70. What is the incidence of atherosclerotic aneurysms?

- >90% affecting abdominal aorta
- Infra-renal segment in 95%
- Male : Female ratio 4:1
- More common in western countries
- 5% over 50s, 15% over 80s
- Associated with iliac aneurysms in 30%
- Associated with popliteal aneurysms in 10%

71. What are the clinical features of abdominal aortic aneurysms?

- Asymptomatic in 75% and found on clinical examination or radiographic
- Central abdominal Pain
- Radiating to the back
- Chronic due to stretching the vessel wall or compression/ erosion of surrounding structures
- Retroperitoneal, Intraperitoneal, abdominal /back/ flank pain due to rupture, shock
- Risk of rupture correlate with aneurysm size
- 5-year rupture rate 25% in AAA >5cm
- High diastolic BP, CAD leads to rupture.

72. What are the causes of vomiting?

Pregnancy, Infectious disease, CNS disorders, opioid, digitalis, GI tract irritation, food poisoning

73. Name the drug therapy for vomiting.

Anti histamine: Promethazine, cyclizine.
Prokinetic: domperidone, metoclopramide.
Serotonin antagonist: Dolasetron, odensetron.
Phinothiazine: Cholrpromazine, perphenazine.

74. Define paroxysmal nocturnal dyspnea.

Attacks of shortness of breath especially at night that awaken the patient.

75. How to measure CVP?

Using one of the proximal lumen or with central venous catheter in the internal jugular or subclavian vein.

76. List down the principles of invasive pressure monitoring.

- Referencing, phlebostasis axis
- Zeroing
- Dynamic response test (square wave test)

77. What are the clinical indications for pulmonary artery catheter?

- ARDS
- Acute respiratory failure
- Cardiac tamponade
- IABP therapy
- Peri-operative infective complication
- Severe shock status

78. What are the long term complications of pulmonary artery catheter?

- Infection
- Sepsis
- Air embolus
- Pulmonary embolism
- Pulmonary infarction and rupture

79. What are complications of AAA rupture?

- Fistulation, rare
- Gut, IVC, left renal vein
- Thrombosis, rare
- Acute lower limb ischaemia
- Distal embolism
- Acute ischaemia to small distal areas (trash foot)
- Distal obliteration
- Claudication, rest pain, gangrene

80. What are the steps of elective surgical

repair done for aneurysms?

- 6-unit cross matched blood
- Mid line or transverse incision
- Aneurysm neck defined and controlled
- Control of normal vessels distal to AAA
- Systemic heparinization, 5000IU
- AAA sac opened and thrombus removed
- Back bleeding from lumber arteries controlled by sutures
- Inlay tube or trouser synthetic graft
- Closure of aneurysm sac over graft

81. What are the steps of emergency surgical repair done for aneurysms?

- Unstable patient, no investigation
- Stable patient, USG/spiral CT
- 10-unit of cross matched blood
- Urinary catheter & 2 large-bore I.V. lines
- Resusitation to systolic BP-100mmHg
- Crash anaesthetic induction
- No heparinization
- Rapid entrance to abdomen & neck control
- If difficult, supra-renal clamp for short period

82. What are the complications of aortic aneurysms surgery?

- Haemorrhage, DIC
- CVA
- Colonic ischaemia, spinal cord ischaemia
- Aorto-enteric fistula
- Graft thrombosis
- Myocardial ischaemia
- Renal failure, ARDS, MODS
- False anastomotic aneurysm
- Distal embolism (trash foot)

83. What are the hemodynamic effects of IABP during inflation and deflation?

- Effects of inflation during diastole
- Increased diastole pressure
- Increased pressure in the aortic root during diastole
- Increased coronary artery perfusion pressure
- Impaired O2 delivery to myocardium

84. What are the complications with IABP therapy?

- Site infection
- Pneumonia
- Arterial trauma
- Thrombo embolism
- Hematologic complication
- Balloon leak or rupture

85. How will you confirm the placement of ET tube?

- End tidal carbon dioxide detection probe placed between BUM & ET tube
- Bilateral chest movement
- Chest x-ray {3-5cm above the carina in adult}
- Position of tube at lip or teeth at 21cm for women 23cm for men

86. What is endovascular repair of aneurysm and what are the complications?

- Patient unfit for surgical repair
- Severe cardio-pulmonary co-morbidities, horse shoe kidney, inflammatory AAA, hostile abdomen.
- Anatomical suitability
- Neck diameter & length
- Iliac arteries diameter & tortuosity
- Morbidity
- Endoleak, migration, kink, thrombosis
- Mortality ~5%
- Flow-up & durability

87. Define heart failure.

- A state in which the heart cannot provide sufficient cardiac output to satisfy the metabolic needs of the body.

- It is commonly termed congestive heart failure (CHF) since symptoms of increased venous pressure are often prominent.

88. What is the etiology of heart failure?

It is a common end point for many diseases of cardiovascular system. **It is caused by:**
Inappropriate work load (volume or pressure overload)
Restricted filling
Myocyte loss

89. What are the causes of left ventricular heart failure?

- **Volume over load:** Regurgitating valve
  – High output status
- **Pressure overload:** Systemic hypertension
  – Outflow obstruction
- **Loss of muscles:** Post MI, Chronic ischemia
  – Connective tissue diseases
  – Infection, Poisons (alcohol, cobalt, doxorubicin)
- **Restricted Filling:** Pericardial diseases, restrictive
  – cardiomyopathy, tachyarrhythmia

90. What are the hemodynamic changes in heart failure?

From hemodynamic stand point HF can be secondary to systolic dysfunction or diastolic dysfunction.

91. What are the neuro hormonal changes in heart failure?

- Increased SNS activity ↑ HR ↑, contractility,
- Vasoconstriction→ ↑® venous return,
- ↑ filling arteriolar constriction →
- After load → ↑ workload
- → ↑ O2 consumption
- ↑Renin-Angiotensin –
- Aldosterone salt & water retention→ ↑ VR and vasoconstriction ↑
- ↑ after load
- ↑ Vasopressin
- ↑ interleukins &TNFa

May have roles in myocyte hypertrophy

- ↑ Endothelin
- Vasoconstriction→ ↑ VR
- ↑ After load

92. What are the physical examination findings in heart failure?

- High diastolic BP & occasional decrease in systolic BP (decapcitated BP), JVD, Rales (Inspiratory)
- Displaced and sustained apical impulses
- Third heart sound – low pitched sound that is heard during rapid filling of ventricle
- Mechanism of S3 sudden deceleration of blood as elastic limits of the ventricles are reached
- Vibration of the ventricular wall by blood filling
- Common in children
- Fourth heart Sound (S4)
- Usually at the end of diastole
- Exact mechanism is not known
- Could be due to contraction of
- atrium against stiff ventricle
- Pale, cold, sweaty skin

93. Discuss Framingham criteria for diagnosis of heart failure.

- **Major Criteria:**
  PND
  JVD
  Rales
  Cardiomegaly
  Acute pulmonary edema

S_3 Gallop
Positive hepatic Jugular reflex
↑ venous pressure > 16 cm H2O

Minor criteria

- Lower limb edema,
- Night cough
- Dyspnea on exertion
- Hepatomegaly
- Pleural effusion
- ↓ vital capacity by 1/3 of normal
- Tachycardia 120 bpm
- Weight loss 4.5 kg over 5 days management

94. What are the nursing responsibilities of patient with artificial airway?

- Maintaining tube placement
- Maintaining proper cuff inflation 22-25 mm of Hg
- Maintaining oxygenation and ventilation
- Maintaining oral care, skin integrity, comfort, communication.

95. What are the indications of mechanical ventilator?

- Hypoxia
- Apnea
- COPD
- Hyperpnoea
- Cardiopulmonary arrest

96. What are indications for ET suctioning?

- Visible secretion in ET
- Sudden onset of respiratory distress
- Suspected aspiration
- Increased peak airway pressure
- Auscultation of adventitious breath sounds
- Decreased PaO2 & SpO2

97. What are the types of mechanical ventilation?

Negative & positive pressure

98. Explain about therapies to treat elevated potassium level?

- Regular IV insulin administration
- Potassium moves into cell when insulin is given
- Sodium bicarbonate
- Therapy can correct acidosis and causes potassium into cell
- Calcium gluconate IV
- Calcium raises the threshold for excitation, resulting in dysrhythmias
- Dialysis
- Heamodialysis can bring potassium level t0 normal with in 30 minutes to 2 hours
- Sodium polystyrene sulfonate (Kayexalate)
- It is mixed in water sorbitol to produce osmotic diarrhea, allowing for evacuation of potassium-rich stool from body.
- Dietary restriction
- Daily potassium intake is limited to 40 mEq

99. What is aneurysm and mention the classification of aneurysms?

- Aneurysms are out pouchings or dilation of the arterial wall and are common problems involving the aorta.

Classification:

- **True aneurysm** – is one in which the wall of the artery form the aneurysm.
- **False aneurysm** – it is not an aneurysm but a disruption of all layers of arterial wall resulting in leaking of blood.

100. What is aortitis?

It is inflammatory disorder with occlusion of the aorta.

101. What is vasculitis?

Vasculitis is a group of disorders characterized by inflammation and necrosis of blood vessel walls.

102. What is thromboangitis obliterans?

It is a vaculities of small and medium sized veins and arteries in the extremities of young adults.

103. What is peripheral arterial disease?

Peripheral arterial disease involves progressive narrowing and degeneration of the arteries of the neck, abdomen and extremities.

104. Write down the indications of negative pressure ventilation.

- Neuromuscular disorder
- CNS disorder
- Severe COPD
- Disease and injuries of spinal cord

105. Define the volume ventilator.

- Volume ventilator
- Predetermined VT is delivered under varying airway pressure.

106. Define the pressure ventilator.

A machine designed to improve the exchange of air between the lungs and the atmosphere.

107. Describe the ventilator setting.

- Respiratory rate: 6-20 b/min
- Tidal volume: 5-15ml/kg
- FiO2: 21% to 100%, PaO2 >60mm of Hg
- SaO2: >90%
- I: E : 1:2 to 1:1.5
- Flow rate: 40 to 100 ml/mt
- Sensitivity trigger: 0.5 – 1cm H2O
- Pressure limit: 10-20 H2O above peak inspiratory pressure.

108. What is the indication of the CMV mode of ventilation?

- Patient with device to breath
- No spontaneous breathing

109. What is assist control mode of ventilation?

To start a patient on assist-control one must select a PEEP (as determined by lung compliance), a minute volume (MV 100ml/kg), a tidal volume (TV 6ml/kg), and a peak flow. The respiratory rate is the MV/TV. The peak flow is usually four times the minute ventilation. The trigger is either set as "flow-by" or a negative pressure of -2cmH2O. Refinement of the settings is determined by the patient's plateau pressure (should be less than 30cmH2O), the patients inspiratory flow demand, and blood gas targets.

110. List down the assessment for valve dysfunction.

Chest pain or discomfort

Weight gain

Prior history of rheumatic heart disease and physical findings of orthopnea

Dyspnea, rales

Pink-tinged sputum

Murmurs

Palpitations

Cyanosis, capillary refill

Edema

Dysrhythmias

111. What is the collaborative management for valvular disorders?

- Nonsurgical management focuses on drug therapy and rest
- Diuretic, beta blockers, digoxin, O2, vasodilators, prophylactic antibiotic therapy
- Manage A-fib, if develops, with conversion if possible, and use of anticoagulation.

112. Write down the risk factors for venous thrombosis.

- Venous stasis
- Damage of the endothelium
- Hypercoagulability of the blood

113. Write about the management of pulmonary embolism.

- Thrombolytic agents
- Intracaval filter
- Pulmonary embolectomy.

114. Mention the complication of pulmonary embolism.

- Pulmonary infarction
- Pulmonary hypertension

115. Write the clinical features of pulmonary embolism?

- Tachypnea or tachycardia
- Cough, pleuritic chest pain
- Hemoptysis, fever
- Sudden changes in mental status
- Anxiety, sudden onset of unexplained dyspnea

116. What is pulmonary embolism?

Pulmonary embolism is the blockage of pulmonary arteries by thrombus, fat or air embolic and tumor tissue.

117. What is a varicose vein?

Varicose veins are dilated, tortuous subcutaneous veins most frequently found in the saphenous system.

118. Write the etiology of varicose veins.

- Congenital weakness of vein structure
- Obesity
- Pregnancy
- Venous obstruction resulting from thrombosis
- Occupations that require prolonged standing

119. List complication of deep vein thrombosis.

- Pulmonary embolism
- Chronic venous insufficiency
- phlegmasia cerulea dolens

120. What is pressure support ventilation?

Pressure support ventilation is the application of positive pressure to the airway only during inspiration.

121. What are indications of critical care?

Patients who are Physiologically unstable, at the risk for life threatening complication and require frequent & invasive monitoring.

122. What are the common problems of critical care patients?

Sepsis, catabolic ARF, Parenteral nutrition, sleep disturbances, sensory perceptional problem, pain, anxiety,
Impaired communication and hyper metabolic state are some of the common problems of critically ill patients.

123. What is the benefit of SIMV mode of ventilation?

- Patient fights ventilator less
- Lower mean airway pressure
- Treatment of muscle atrophy

124. What are the disadvantages of SIMV?

Dependent on patients' spontaneous breathing. Low SIMV may lead to a drop in the oxygen saturation.

125. What are the pathophysiological changes and signs and symptoms of aortic stenosis?

- Valve becomes stiff and fibrotic, impeding blood flow with LV contraction, LV hypertrophy, increased O2 demands and pulmonary congestion
- **Causes** – Rheumatic fever, congenital, arthrosclerosis and calcification in the elderly

- **Complications** – Right sided heart failure, pulmonary edema, and A-fib
- **S/S – Early**: dyspnea, angina, syncope
- **Late**: marked fatigue, debilitation and peripheral cyanosis, crescendo-decrescendo murmur is heard

126. What are the pathophysiological changes and signs and symptoms of aortic regurgitation?

- Aortic valve leaflets do not close properly during diastole
- The valve ring that attaches to the leaflets may be dilated, loose or deformed
- The ventricle dilates to accommodate the blood volume and hypertrophies
- Causes: Infective endocarditis, congenital, hypertension, Marfan's
- signs and symptoms are dyspnea, orthopnea, palpitations and angina
- systolic pressure with bounding pulse
- high pitch, blowing, decrescendo diastolic murmur.

127. List down the clinical manifestations of hypokalemia.

- Generalized muscle weakness
- Fatigue
- Diminished or absent reflexes
- Decreased GI motility
- Anorexia
- Abdominal distension
- Paralytic ileus
- Drowsiness
- Irritability
- Tetany
- Coma.

128. Enlist the clinical manifestations of hyperkalemia.

- Impaired muscle activity
- Weakness
- Muscle pain/ cramps
- Increased GI motility
- Nausea
- Diarrhea
- Oliguria
- Dizziness
- Irritability

129. List interventions for constipation.

- Laxatives-Senna, bisacodyl etc
- Stool softeners
- Enemas
- Position
- Exercise

130. What are the indications of VAD therapy?

The target patients for this therapy fall into three possible intentions of treatment or indications of VAD placement:

BTT, for patients who are transplant candidates but who will not survive waiting until an organ is available

DT, for patients who are not transplant candidates

BTR, for patients in whom the native heart function may possibly be recovered

131. List relative contra indication of VAD.

- BSA less than 1.5M2
- Renal or liver failure.
- Comorbidities that could limit life expectancy to less than 3 years.

132. Mention the complications of VAD.

- Bleeding
- Cardiac tamponade
- Ventricular fibrillation
- Infection
- Arrhythmias
- Renal failure

133. What are the premedication of ET tube

intubation?

- Midazolam – sedative hypnotics
- Fentanyl-decrease pain of laryngospasmano intubation
- Succinyl-chloride-skeletal muscle paralysis
- Atropine-limit the secretion

134. What are the types of valvular heart disease?

- Mitral Stenosis
- Mitral Regurgitation
- Mitral valve prolapse
- Aortic stenosis
- Aortic regurgitation
- Tricuspid stenosis
- Tricuspid regurgitation

135. What are the signs and symptoms of Rheumatic heart disease?

- Subjective symptoms
- Prior history of rheumatic fever
- General malaise
- Pain – may or may not be present
- Objective symptoms
- Temperature
- Murmurs
- Dyspnea
- polyarthritis

136. Mention the correction of reversible causes of heart failure.

- Diet : Salt & fluid restriction
- Mild diuretics and loop diuretics
- Pottassium sparing diuretics
- ACE inhibitors
- Beta blockers
- Vasodilators
- Positive inotropic agents
- Anticoagulation (coumadin)
- Implantable ventricular assist devices
- Biventricular pacing (artificial heart)

Test Series VI

1. **Write about the general manifestations of disorder of urinary system?**
Fatigue, headache, blurred vision, elevated blood pressure, excessive thirst, cognitive change, anorexia, nausea & vomiting, chills, itching, change in body weight.
2. **Explain the criteria for the diagnosis of interstitial cystitis/ painful bladder syndrome.**
I. Inclusion Criteria
   - Pain during bladder filling that is relieved by voiding
   - Bother some urinary urgency and frequency
   - Small bladder capacity or urodynamic testing.
   - Cystoscopic evidence of ulcerations or glomerulation

   II Exclusion criteria
   - bladder capacity >350ml on urodynamic testing
   - Overactive bladder contractions on urodynamic testing.
   - Active genital herpes
3. **Write about ileal conduit.**
Ureters are implanted into part of ileum or colon that has been from intestinal tract abdominal stoma is created.
Advantage: Relatively good urine flow with few physiologic alterations.
Disadvantage: External appliance necessary to continually collect urine.
Special Considerations:
   - Surgical procedure is more complex
   - Postoperative complication may be increased
   - Reabsorption of urea by illeum occurs
   - Meticulous attention is necessary to care for stoma & collecting devices.
4. **What is addisonian crisis?**
A life threatening disorder caused by adrenal hormone insufficiency. It is precipitated by infection, trauma, stress, or surgery. Death can occur from shock, vascular collapse, or hyperkalemia.
5. **What is HHNS?**
HHNS is hyperglycemic hyperosmolar nonketotic syndrome. Extreme hyperglycemia without acidosis. Usually occurs in type 2 diabetes mellitus when diabetes is uncontrolled or undiagnosed or during stress or infection.
6. **What are all the clinical manifestations related to the urinary system?**
Edema: Facial, ankle, ascites, anasarca, sacral
Pain: Dysuria, flank or costo, vertebral

angle, groin, suprapubic.

Pattern of urination: Frequency, urgency, retention, dysuria, nocturia, overactive bladder, incontinence, dribbling, urine output,-anuria, oliguria, polyuria.

7. Describe about the stages of chronic kidney disease.

Stages	Description	GFR	Action
Risk Period	At increased risk for CKD	[ml/ min/1.73m2] ≥ 90 [with CKD risk factor]	Screening CKD risk reduction
Stage 1	Kidney damage with normal (or) increased GFR	≥ 90	Diagnosis & treatment of comorbid condition CVD risk reduction
Stage 2	Kidney damage with mild decreased GFR	60-89	Estimate of progression
Stage 3	Moderate decreased GFR	30-59	Evaluation and treatment of complications
Stage 4	Severe decreased GFR	15-29	Preparation for renal replacement therapy
Stage 5	Kidney failure	<15 or dialysis	Renal replacement

8. Describe the collaborative care for acute glomerulonephritis

I Diagnostic

- History and physical examination
- Urinalysis
- CBC with WBC differential
- Bun, serum creatinine, & albumin
- Renal biopsy (If indicated)

II Collaborative Therapy

- Rest
- Sodium & fluid restriction
- Diuretics Antihypertensive therapy Adjustment of dietary Protein intake to level of proteinuria and uremia.

9. Explain about cutaneous ureterostomy.

- Ureters are excised from bladder and brought through abdominal wall and stoma is created
- Ureteral stoma may be created from both ureters (or) ureters may be brought together and one stoma created.
- **Advantage:** No need for major surgery as required with ileal conduct
- **Disadvantage:** External appliance necessary because or continuous urine drainage, possibility of stricture or stenosis of small stoma
- **Stomal consideration:** Periotic catheterizations may be required to dilate stomas to maintain patency.

10. Mechanism of renal osteo dystrophy.

- Decreased PO2 excretion
- Decreased GFR
- Kidney failure
- Activation of vitamin D
- Impaired calcium absorption from gut
- Decreased serum calcium
- Increased PTH → osteitis fibrosa
- Bone demineralization→osteomalacia
- Increased serum ca, po4, metastatic calcification

11. Describe diagnostic studies of urinary system and nursing responsibility.

BUN – Commonly used to identify presence of renal problems. Concentration of urea in blood is regulated by rate at which kidney excretes urea.

Normal finding:10-30mg/dl

Nursing responsibility:

Explain test and watch for postpuncture bleeding. Be aware that, when interpreting BUN, non renal factors may cause increase in rapid cell destruction from infection, fever, GI bleeding, trauma, antibiotic activity and excessive muscle break down, corticosteroid therapy.

12. What is creatinine?

Creatinine is more reliable than bun as a determinant of renal function. creatinine is end product of muscle and protein metabolism and is caliberated as a constant rate. Normal Finding: 0.5-1.5 mg/dl results are higher in men.

Nursing Responsibility-Postpuncture bleeding.

13. What is Intravenous Pyelogram (IVP)?

In Intravenous pyelogram, x-ray examination visualizes urinary position, size, and shape as the kidney, ureters, and bladder can be evaluated. Cysts, tumors, lesions, and obstructions causes a distortion in the normal appearance of these structures, patient with significantly decreased renal function should not have IVP because contrast media can be nephrotoxic and worsen renal function.

14. Name common microorganisms causing urinary tract infections.

Escherichia coli, pseudomonas, enterococcus, staphylococcus, klebsiella, serratica, enterobacter, candida albicans, proteus.

15. Explain the medical terminology in urinary system

Pyelonephritis: Pyelonephritis implies inflammation of the renal parenchyma and collecting system.

Cystitis: Cystitis indicates inflammation of the bladder wall

Urethritis: Urethritis means inflammation of the Urethra

Urosepsis: Urosepsis is a urinary tract infection that has spread into the systemic circulation and is a life threatening condition requiring emergency treatment.

16. What are the predisposing factor to urinary tract infections?

- Urinary tract calculi
- Catheters
- Urinary tract instrumentation
- Congenital defects leading to obstruction or urinary stasis
- Fistula exposing urinary stream to skin, vagina or fecal steam.
- Shorter female urethra and colonization from normal vagina flora
- Obesity

17. Describe collaborative care for acute pyelonephritis.

- Empirically selected broad-spectrum antibiotics for eg.; Ampicillin, vancomycin
- Combined with aminoglycoside. (Eg: tobramycin, gentamicin)
- Switch to sensitivity – Guided therapy. (Eg: trimethoprim-sulfamethoxazole) when results of urine and blood culture are available.
- Fluoroquinolones. (Eg: ciprofloxacin, ofloxacin, norfloxacin, gatifloxacin)
- Adequate fluid intake
- Nonsteroidal anti inflammatory drugs and antipyretic drugs.
- Followup urine culture and imaging studies.

18. What are causes of nephrotic syndrome?

Primary glomerular disease.
Extrarenal causes (Multisystem disease)
Infections
Neoplasms
Allergens (Eg: Pollen)
Drugs (Penicillin, NSAIDS).

19. Write about the risk factors for the development of urinary tract calculi.

i) Metabolic

Abnormalities that result in increased urine level of calcium, Oxaluric acid, uric acid, or citric acid.

ii) Climate

Warm climate that cause increase fluid loss, low urine volume, and increased solute concentration in urine

iii) Diet

Large intake or dietary proteins that increases uric acid excretion excessive amount of tea or fruit juices that elevate urinary oxalate level

Large intake of calcium 4 oxalate

Low fluid intake that increases urinary concentration

iv) Genetic factors -Family history of stone formation

Cystinuria

Renal acidosis

v) Life style-Sedentary occupation, immobility

20. List out the types of urinary incontinence.

- Stress incontinence
- Urge incontinence
- Over flow incontinence
- Reflex incontinence
- Incontinence after trauma (or) surgery
- Functional Incontinence.

21. List down the interventions for urinary Incontinence.

- Life style modification
- Smoking cessation
- Weight reduction
- Good bowel regimen
- Reduction of bladder irritants such as
- caffeine
- Fluid modification

22. What is the pelvic floor muscle?

Pelvic floor muscle provides support for bladder and rectum and in women, the vagina the uterus. If it weakens or is damaged, it cannot support these organs and their position can change.

This causes problems with the normal bladder and rectal function. For weak pelvic floor muscle, want to do special muscle stronger, prevent unwanted urine leakage & lesson urinary urgency.

23. How to do the pelvic floor exercise?

There are two kinds of exercise

i) Short squeezes

ii) Long squeezes

i) Short squeezes: It tightens the pelvic floor muscle quickly, squeeze hard for 2 seconds, and then relax the muscle also strong urinary urges.

Try to tighten your pelvic floor muscle quickly and hard several times in a day until the urge passes

ii) Long squeezes: It is tighten the muscle for 5 to 10 sec before you relax. Do both of these exercises 40 to 40 time each day

24. Whart are the indications for urinary catheterizations?

- Relief of urinary retention caused by lower urinary tract obstruction, paralysis, or inability to void
- Bladder decompression
- Facilitation of surgical repair of urethra and surrounding structure.
- Splinting of ureters or urethra to fa-

cilitate healing after surgery or other trauma in area
- To measure the accurate rate of urinary output
- Measurement of residual urine after urination if portable ultrasound not available.
- Terminal illness or severe impairment, which make positioning or clothing changes uncomfortable (or) which is associated with intractable pain.

25. List down the nursing intervention of suprapubic catheters.
- Prevent dislodgement of catheter
- Care of the tube of catheter is similar to that of the urethral catheter
- A pectin-base skin barrier is effective around the insertion site in protecting the skin from backdown
- Preventing tube kinking by coiling the excess tubing and maintaining gravity drainage
- Having the patient turn from side to side
- Milking the tube.

26. Define Nephrostomy.

Catheter is inserted into pelvis of kindney, procedure may be done to one or both kidneys and may be temporary or permanent. It is most frequently done in advanced disease as palliative procedure.

Advantage: No need for major surgery

Disadvantage: High risk of renal infection
- Predisposition to calculus formation from catheter.
- Special Considerations
- Nephrostomy tube may have to be changed every month, catheter must never be clamped

27. What are prerenal cause of acute renal failure.

Hypovolemia
Decreased cardiac out put
Decreased peripheral vascular resistance
Decreased renovascular blood flow

28. List out intrarenal cause of acute renal failure.

Prolonged prerenal ischemia
Nephrotoxic injury
Interstitial nephritis
Acute glomerulonephritis
Thrombotic disorders
Malignant hypertension
Systemic lupus erythematus

29. List postrenal causes of renal failure.
- Benign prostatic hyperplasia
- Bladder cancer
- Calculi formation
- Neuromuscular disorder
- Prostate cancer
- Spinal cord disease
- Strictures
- Trauma (back, pelvis, perineum)

30. Define dialysis and list out the types.

Dialysis is the movement of fluid and molecules across a semipermeable membrane from one compartment to another

2 types are there
1) Peritoneal dialysis
2) Hemodialysis dialysis

31. Define about peritoneal dialysis and hemodialysis.

In Peritoneal dialysis, the peritoneal membrane acts as the semipermeable membrane. hemodialysis. In HD artificial membrane (usually made of cellulose based or synthetic materials) is used as the semipermeable membrane and is in contact with the patient's blood.

32. What is trousseau's sign?

A sign found in hypocalcemia. Carpal spasm can be elicited by compressing the upper arm and causing ischemia to the nerves distally.

33. Explain the comparison of prerenal oliguria with oliguria of acute renal failure.

Characteristics	Prerenal oliguria	Oliguria of acute renal failure
1. Urine output	Low	Low
2. BUN	Elevated	Elevated
3. Serum creatinine	Normal (or) Slightly elevated	Elevated
4. Urine Specific gravity	High	at 1-010
5. Urine Sodium	Low	High

34. Define continuous ambulatory peritoneal dialysis.

CAPD is carried out manually by exchanging 1.5 to 3 (usually 2L) of peritoneal dialysate at least 4 times daily, with dwelling times of 4 to 10 hours.

Eg: One schedule starts the exchanges at 7am, 12 noon, 5pm and 10 pm. In this procedure the person instills 2 L of dialysate from a collapsible plastic bag into the peri toneal cavity through a disposable plastic tube.

35. Describe contraindications for peritoneal dialysis.

- History of multiple abdominal surgical procedure (or) chronic abdominal pathologic condition (eg. Pancreatitis, diverticulitis, recurrent abdominal wall (or) inguinal hernia obesity with large abdominal wall & fat deposits
- Pre existing vertebral disease (Eg. chronic back problem)
- Severe obstructive pulmonary disease.

36. Explain the advantages and disadvantages of peritoneal dialysis.

Advantages	Disadvantages
i) Immediate initiation	Bacterial (or) Chemical peritonitis
ii) Less complicated	Protein loss into dialysate
iii) Portable system with CAPD	Exit site & tunnel infections
iv) Fever dietary restrictions	Hyperglycenia
v) Relatively short training time	Aggravated hyperlipidemia
vi) Less cardiovascular stress	Specially trained personal needed catheter can migrate

37. List out complication of peritoneal dialysis.

- Exit site infection
- Peritonitis
- Abdominal Pain
- Outflow problem
- Hernias
- Lower back problems
- Bleeding
- Pulmonary complications
- Carbohydrate & lipid abnormalities
- Encapsulations sclerosing peritonitis and loss of ultrafiltration

38. Name complications arising out of hemodialysis.

- Hypotension
- Muscle Cramps
- Loss of blood

- Hepatits
- Sepsis
- Disuse Syndrome
- Malignancies
- Recurrence of original renal disease
- Corticosteriod related complication

39. Explain about therapies to treat elevated potassium level.

- Regular insulin administration-IV
- Sodium bicarbonate
- Calcium gluconate-IV
- Dialysis
- Sodium polystrene sulfonate (Kayeralate)
- Dietary Restriction

40. What are the extrarenal causes of glomerulo nephritis?

- Multisystem disease
- Systemic lupus erythematosus
- Diabetes mellitus
- Amyloidosis

41. Describe the comparison of hemodialysis.

Advantages	Disadvantage
Rapid fluid removal	Vascular access problems
Rapid removal of urea & creatinine	Dietary & fluid restriction
Effective potassium removal, less protein loss	Extensive equipment necessary
Lowering of serum triglycerides	Hypotension during dialysis

42. What are the types of primary glomerular disease?

- Membranous proliferative glomerulonephritis
- Primary nephrotic syndrome
- Focal glomerulonephritis
- Inherited nephrotic disease.

Test Series VII

1. **What is Addisonian crisis?**
   A life threatening disorder caused by adrenal hormone insufficiency. It is precipitated by infection, trauma, stress, or surgery. Death can occur from shock, vascular collapse, or hyperkalemia.
2. **What is HHNS?**
   HHNS is hyperglycemic hyperosmolar nonketotic syndrome. Extreme hyperglycemia without acidosis. Usually occurs in type 2 diabetes mellitus when diabetes is uncontrolled or undiagnosed, or during stress or infection.
3. **What are the disorders of pituitary gland?**
   Hyperpituitarism
   Acromegaly
   Cushings syndrome
   Hypopituitarism
   Posterior pituitary diabetes insipidus
   SIADH (Syndrome of inappropriate antidiuretpormone)
   Pickardt-Fahlbusch-Syndrome
   Sheehans syndrome
4. **What are disorders of adrenal glands?**
   Adrenal cortex
   Addison's disease
   Cushing's syndrome
   Aldosteronism (Conn's syndrome)
   Adrenal medulla
   Pheochromocytoma.
5. **What is Addison's disease?**
   Hyposecretion of adrenal cortex hormones (glucocorticoids and mineralocorticoids) from the adrenal gland, resulting in deficiency of the steroid hormones. The condition is fatal if left untreated.
6. **What is hypophysectomy?**
   The removal of the pituitary gland is known as hypophysectomy.
7. **What are disorders of the thyroid gland?**
   - Hypothyroidism (Myxedema)
   - Hyperthyroidism (Graves' disease)
8. **What is adrenalectomy?**
   The surgical removal of an adrenal gland. Lifelong steroid replacement is necessary with a bilateral adrenalectomy. Temporary steroid replacement, up to 2 years, is necessary for a unilateral adrenalectomy.
9. **What is Chvostek's sign?**
   A spasm of the facial muscles elicited by tapping the facial nerve in the region of the parotid gland. It is noted in hypocalcemia.
10. **What is cushing's syndrome?**
    A condition resulting from the hypersecretion of glucocorticoids from the adrenal cortex.

11. What is dawn phenomenon?

Results from a nocturnal release of growth hormone, which may cause blood glucose elevations about 3 am. Treatment includes administering an evening dose of intermediate acting insulin at 10 p.m.

12. What is diabetic ketoacidosis?

A complication of diabetes mellitus that develops when a severe insulin deficiency occurs. DKA is a life threatening condition. Hyperglycemia that progress to ketoacidosis occurs.

13. What is diabetes mellitus?

A chronic and potentially disabling disease characterized by elevated blood glucose levels. A chronic disorder of glucose intolerance and impaired carbohydrate, protein and lipid metabolism caused by a deficiency of insulin results in hyperglycemia.

14. What is Graves' disease?

Graves' disease (hyperthyroidism) is known as thyrotoxicosis. A hyperthyroid state resulting from hypersecretion of thyroid hormone.

15. What is insulin waning?

A progressive rise in the blood glucose level from bedtime to morning. Treatment includes increasing the evening (predinner or bedtime) dose of intermediate or long-acting insulin, or instituting a dose of insulin before the evening meal if one is not already prescribed.

16. What is myxedema?

A hypothyroid state resulting from a hyposecretion of thyroid hormone. The condition occurs in adulthood.

17. What is trousseau's sign?

A sign found in hypocalcemia. Carpal spasm can be elicited by compressing the upper arm and causing ischemia to the nerves distally.

18. What is thyroid storm?

An acute and fatal thyroid hormone into the bloodstream. It can also occur as a result of severe infection and stress.

19. What is myxedema coma?

A rare but serious disorder that results from persistently low thyroid production. It can be precipitated by acute illness, rapid withdrawal of thyroid medication, anesthesia and surgery, hypothermia and the use of sedatives and narcotics.

20. What is Somogyi's phenomenon?

A rebound phenomenon that occurs during the initial period of serum glucose control. It develops at peak insulin times and during the night. Normal or elevated blood glucose levels are present at bedtime, a decrease occurs at about 2 to 3 a.m. to hypoglycemic levels and a subsequent increase occurs as a result of the production of counterregulatory hormones.

21. What are all the risk factors for endocrine disorders?

- Hereditary
- Congenital
- Trauma
- Environmental
- Secondary to other disorders.

22. What are the signs of tetany?

- Positive Chvostek's sign
- Positive Trousseau's sign
- Wheezing and dyspnea
- Dysphagia
- Numbness and tingling of the face and extremities
- Carpopedal spasm
- Visual disturbances (photophobia)
- Muscle and abdominal cramps
- Cardiac dysrhythmias
- Seizures.

23. What is pheochromocytoma?
A catecholomine producing tumor usually found in the adrenal gland but also may be found in the abdomen.

24. What is hyperaldosteronism (Conn's syndrome)?
A hypersecretion of aldosterone (mineralocorticoids) from the adrenal cortex of the adrenal gland. Most commonly caused by an adenoma.

25. What are complications of insulin therapy?
- Local allergic reactions
- Insulin lipodystrophy
- Insulin resistance
- Dawn phenomenon
- Somogyi's phenomenon
- Insulin waning

26. What are symptoms of diabetes mellitus?
- Polyuria
- Polydipsia
- Polyphagia
- Hyperglycemia
- Weight loss
- Blurred vision
- Slow wound healing
- Weakness and paresthesias.

27. What are functions of endocrine glands?
- Maintenance and regulation of vital functions
- Response to stress and injury
- Growth and development
- Energy metabolism
- Reproduction
- Fluid, electrolyte, and acid-base balance.

28. What are all endocrine glands?
- Pituitary gland
- Adrenal gland
- Thyroid gland
- Parathyroid gland
- Pancreas
- Ovaries
- Testes

29. What are risk factors for endocrine disorders?
- Hereditary
- Congenital
- Trauma
- Environmental
- Secondary to other disorders.

30. What are functions of endocrine glands?
- Maintenance and regulation of vital functions
- Response to stress and injury
- Growth and development
- Energy metabolism
- Reproduction
- Fluid, electrolyte, acid-base balance.

31. What are complications of insulin therapy?
- Local allergic reactions
- Insulin lipodystrophy
- Insulin resistance
- Dawn phenomenon
- Somogyi's phenomenon
- Insulin waning

32. What is hypophysectomy?
The removal of the pituitary gland is known as hypophysectomy.

33. Describe problems due to dysfunction of the hypothalamus-pituitary-ovarian axis?
- Oligomenorrhea is a HPO disorder associated with infertility.
- Irregular menstrual cycles that fluctuate from 35 days to 2-5 months
- DUB or prolonged periods of breakthrough bleeding.
- Hyperandrogenism, acne, hirsutism, and baldness, obesity and decreased fertility in polycystic ovarian syndrome.

Test Series VIII

1. **Define BPH.**
   The term refers to the new growth of epithelial cells, especially stromal elements in the prostate gland.
2. **Define hypospadias.**
   The urethral meatus is located in the ventral surface of the penis anywhere from the corona to the perineum.
3. **Define varicocele.**
   It is the dilation of the veins that drain the testes. Mostly located in the left side of the scrotum. Treatment is done by injection of sclerosing agent or by ligation of the spermatic cord.
4. **List clinical manifestations of BPH.**
   diminution in the caliber and force of the urinary stream, hesitancy in initiating voiding, dribbling at the end of the urination, a feeling of incomplete bladder emptying because of urinary retention, nocturia, dysuria and urgency.
5. **Define testicular torsion.**
   It involves a twisting of the spermatic cord that supplies the blood to the testes and epididymis. It is most commonly seen in puberty.
6. **List down the invasive treatment of BPH.**
   - Trans urethral ultra sound guided laser induced prostatectomy (TULIP)
   - Trans urethral resection of prostate (TURP)
   - Tran urethral incision of prostate (TUIP)
   - Supra pubic resection of prostate
   - Retropubic resection of prostate
   - Perineal resection of prostate
7. **Mention the complications of BPH.**
   - Urinary tract infection
   - Calculi formation
   - Hematuria
   - Hydroureter
   - Hydroneohrosis
   - Pyelonephritis
8. **Describe post operative care after prostatectomy.**
   - Continuous bladder irrigation for 24 hours
   - Maintain intake output chart
   - Fluid intake 2000-3000ml/day
   - Watch for signs of infection
   - Prevent constipation
   - Avoid heavy lifting (10 pounds)
   - Refrain from driving or intercourse for 6 weeks after surgery.
9. **Write the chemotherapeutic drugs for testicular cancer.**

Bleomycin, vincristine, cisplatin, vinblastin

10. Define vasectomy.
It is the bilateral surgical ligation or resection of the vasdeferens performed for the purpose of sterilization.

11. List management for Ca prostate.
TURP, total prostatectomy, radiation therapy, hormonal manipulation (estrogen, luteinizing – releasing), radiation therapy, chemotherapy.

12. Define circumcision.
It is the removal of foreskin of the penis, may be done for religious, cultural, or hygienic reasons.

13. List complications of prostatectomy.
Hemorrhage, infection, bladder spasm and erectile problems.

14. What are the risk factors of prostate carcinoma?
Sexual activity, socioeconomic class, alcohol use, family history, high fat diet and environmental factors.

15. Name metastatic sites of prostatic cancer.
Pelvic lymph nodes, bones, bladder, lungs and liver.

16. List the clinical manifestations of Ca prostate.
Dysuria, hesitancy, dribbling, frequency, urgency, hematuria, nocturia and retention, hard and unilateral enlargement of prostate, pain in lumbosacral area.

17. Define phimosis.
The fore skin constricting around the opening and making retraction difficult. It is caused by edema and inflammation of the foreskin.

18. Define priapism.
It is a painful erection, lasting longer than 6 hours and unable to urinate.
Causes – Thrombosis of corpora cavernosa, leukemia, sickle cell anemia.

19. Define cryptorchidism.
It is the undescended testis, most common congenital testicular condition.

20. What is meant by DES sons?
DES sons refer to the male children born to women who took diethylstilbestrol during pregnancy. Born with undescended testis.

21. Define hydrocele.
A hydrocele results from interference with lymphatic drainage of the scrotum, with swelling of tunica vaginalis that surrounds the testis.

22. Name tumor markers of testicular cancer.
Alpha feto protein, human chorionic gonadotropin.

23. What are medical treatments for BPH?
Intermittent or indwelling catheterization, high fluid intake, antibiotics, alpha adrenergic blockers, finastride therapy, balloon dilatation.

24. Define PSA.
Prostate Specific Antigen-A glycoprotein that is detected only in the epithelial cells of the prostate.

25. What are the causes of infertility in male?
Pre testicular and endocrine causes

- Testicular causes
- Post testicular causes-infection, obstruction or vasaectomy

26. Mention diagnostic investigations for BPH.
Urine analysis, serum creatinine and BUN, prostatic specific antigen, urodynamic flow studies, transurethral ultrasound and cystoscopy.

27. What are all the causes of prostitis?
Bacteria, viruses, sudden decrease in sexual activity

28. List down the management of prostitis.
Long term administration of antibiotics, anti-inflammatory agent, frequent prostatic massage, sitz bath and stool softners.

Test Series IX

1. **Define ecchymosis.**
   Large bruise like lesion caused by collection of extra vascular blood in dermis and subcutaneous tissue caused due trauma and bleeding disorders.
2. **Enlist the treatment for psoriasis.**
   - Topical corticosteroids
   - Tar and anthralin
   - UV light with or without psoralen
   - Systemic antimetabolites (methotrexate)
   - immunosuppressants (cyclosporine) IV or IM
   - Retinoid
   - Infliximab
3. **List down the danger signals suggestive of malignant transformation of moles.**
   - Change in color
   - Change in diameter
   - Change in outline
   - Change in surface characteristics(scale, erosion)
   - Change in consistency (softening)
   - Change in symptoms (pruritus)
   - Change in shape
   - Change in surrounding skin
4. **How do we predict skin breakdown?**
   - Impaired sensory perception
   - Moisture
   - Decreased level
5. **What is meant by erythema?**
   Redness occurring in patches of variable in size and shape due to heat exposure, drugs, alcohol, UV rays.
6. **List the fungal infections of the skin.**
   - Tinea corporis
   - Tinea cruris
   - Tinea unguium
   - Tinea pedis
   - Candidiasis
7. **List down the types of skin carcinoma.**
   - Basal cell carcinoma
   - Squamous cell carcinoma
   - Malignant melanoma
   - Cutaneous T cell lymphoma
   - Kaposi's sarcoma
8. **List down the nursing action to prevent skin breakdown.**
   - Assess the skin breakdown
   - Change the position every 2 hours and give back care
   - Pat dry the skin
   - Advice balanced diet
   - Active and passive exercise
   - Early ambulation

9. Define lichenification.

Thickening of skin with accentuated skin markings due to repeated skin scratching, rubbing and irritation.

10. What is meant by telangiectasia?

Visibly dilated, superficial, cutaneous small blood vessels, commonly found on face and thighs due to aging, acne, sun exposure, alcohol, liver failure, radiation and skin tumor.

11. Define intertrigo.

Dermatitis of overlying surfaces of the skin caused due to moisture, irritation, obesity, candida infection.

Treatment-Promoting drying, aeration, loose fitting cloths, periodical removal of clothes to dry.

12. Define petechiae.

Pinpoint, discrete deposit of blood less than 1-2 mm in the extra articular tissues and visible through the skin or mucous membrane caused due to inflammation, marked dilation, blood vessel trauma, blood dyscrasias that results in bleeding tendencies.

13. Define pseudofolliculitis.

It is an inflammatory response to an ingrown hair that is thought to occur after shaving closely, and is characterized by pustules and papules.

14. What is keloid and mangolian spots?

Keloid: Over growth of collagenous tissue at site of the skin injury. It is a benign outgrowth.

Mangolian spot: It is a benign bluish – black macules.

15. Define actinic keratosis.

It is also known as solar keratosis; consist of hyperkeratotic papules and plaques occurring on skin exposed areas. It is a malignant form of squamous cell carcinoma occurring in older white population.

Treatment: Cryosurgery, 5FU, retinol-A, laser resurfacing

16. What are the types of melanoma?

- Superficial spreading melanoma
- Lentigo malignant melanoma
- Acral-lentiginous melanoma
- Nodular melanoma

17. List down the plastic surgeries for dermatologic problems.

- Elective cosmetic surgery
- Chemical face lift
- Topical tretinoin
- Alpha hydroxy acid
- Dermabrasion
- Botulinum toxin injection
- Face lift
- Liposuction
- Skin grafts

18. What are the types of skin grafts?

- Autografts (from the patients own body)
- Isografts (from an identical twin
- Allografts (from the same species)
- Xenografts (from the other species)

19. What is skin flap?

Moving a section of skin and subcutaneous tissue from, one part of the body to another without terminating the vascular attachment (pedicle).

20. What is soft tissue expansion?

It is a technique for providing skin for resurfacing a defect, such as a burn scar for removing a disfiguring mark. A subcutaneous tissue expander placed under the skin in OP or weekly expansion with saline solution at home is done for 3-4 months until it reaches the desired size and the expanded flap is used as an advancement flap.

21. What are the types of dermatitis?
- Contact dermatitis – due to allergens
- Nummular eczema-coin shaped oozing crusting patches
- Atopic dermatitis-due to asthma
- Irritant dermatitis
- Sebborrheic dermatitis
- Stasis dermatitis

22. Name bacterial infections of the skin.
- Impetigo
- Folliculitis
- Furuncle
- Carbuncle
- Cellulitis

23. What are the causes of skin cancer?
- Excessive skin exposure
- Radiation
- Scars and some types of nevi
- Genetic skin type

24. Difference between basal cell carcinoma and squamous cell carcinoma.

S. no	Basal cell carcinoma	Squamous cell carcinoma
1	Nodular and ulcerative type with pearly white border	Firm nodules with or with out ulcer, a cutaneous, indurated plaque
2.	Occur in sun exposed area	Occur in previously damaged skin, radiation or scar
3.	Never metastize	Infiltrate/ metastize to surrounding cells

25.Define nikolsky's sign

It is positive in pemphigus vulgaris. When the epidermis can be rubbed off by slight friction or injury, even a slight pressure on an intact blister may cause it to spread to adjacent skin.

26. List down the management for herpes simplex.
- Analgesics
- Antiviral drug
- Avoiding exposure to sunlight
- Frequent handwashing
- Not pricking at lesions
- Avoiding sexual intercourse, kissing,not sharing lipstick

27. Define banking skin.

Skin grafts can be removed and harvested and stored for application later. It is folded in a dermis to dermis pattern to preserve moisture and then wrapped in a moist saline gauze, impregnated with petrolatum and kept in air tight environment at 4 degree celcius for 10-20 days.

28. List down type of skin flap.
- Axial skin flap
- Muscle flap plus skin graft
- Free flap
- Mucocutaneous flap
- Omental flap

29. Define cryosurgery.

Cryosurgery is using liquid nitrogen in cotton tipped applicator or spraying device to destroy the growth. No local anaesthesia is required.

30. List down the signs of pressure ulcer.
- Areas of skin redness
- Development of foul odor or drainage
- Check the warmth
- Blister formation

31. Write about debridement for the pressure ulcer.
- Sharp debridement
- Mechanical debridement
- Enzymatic debridement
- Autolytic debridement

32. List down the medical management for acne vulgaris.

- Benzoyl peroxide – To decrease the sebum production
- Vitamin A (Tretinoin) – Clears the keratin plug from pilosebaceous ducts
- Topical antibiotics – Tetracycline, clindamicin, erythromycin
- Systemic antibiotics
- Oral retinoids
- Hormone therapy (estrogen)

33. List down the management for scabies.

- Application of lindane, crotamiton, 5% permothin after warm soapy bath
- Dry in hot sun for 12-24 hours and wash with hot water and dry clean
- Repeat after one week
- Oral corticosteroids, antihistamines
- Treat family members
- Wash cloths separately and use separate soap and towel
- Treat coexisting STD and pediculosis

34. Define stasis dermatitis.

It is characterized by development of areas of very dry skin and sometimes shallow ulcers in the lower legs due to venous insufficiency.

35. How do you manage for stasis dermatitis?

- Leg elevation
- Wearing support hose/ elastic wrap
- Refraining from cross leg
- Walking instead of standing and calf exercise
- Moisture retention dressing
- Unna boots and gradient pressure wraps.

36. Define bullous impetigo.

It is a deep seated skin infection caused by Staphylococcus aureus. It is characterized by bullae (large fluid filled blisters) occurring on exposed areas of body, face, neck and extremities.

37. List down the clinical manifestations of herpes zoster.

- Painful vesicular eruptions preceded by pain along the area of distribution of sensory nerves
- Unilateral distribution band like configuration confined to face and trunk
- Eye pain if ophthalmic nerve is involved

Test Series X

1. **What is osteomalacia?**

   Osteomalecia is a metabolic disease characterized by inadequate nutrition of bone because of the mineralization there is softening and wakening of the skeleton causing pain, tenderness to touch, bowing of the bone and pathologic fracture.

2. **List out risk factors of osteoporosis.**
   - Advanced age
   - Female gender
   - Thin, small framed
   - Family history of osteoporosis
   - Diet low in calcium
   - Excessive use of alcohol
   - Excess caffeine use
   - Low testosterone level

4. **Define kyphosis.**

   Osteoporosis occurs most commonly in the bone of the spine, hips and wrists overtime weakening and fracture of the vertebrae produce a gradual loss of height and a humped back down.

5. **Enlist principles of fracture healing.**
   - Fracture hematoma
   - Granulation tissue
   - Callus formation
   - Ossification
   - Consolidation
   - Remodeling

6. **What is paget's disease?**

   Paget's (ostectes deformans) is a metabolic bone disorder affecting normal bone remodeling. Synchronized breakdown of older bone and formation of new bone. When unsynchronized remodeling occurs, there is increased breakdown and formation of bone the results in enlarged, abnormally formed and brittle bone. Most commonly affecting the skull, femur, tibia, pelvic bones and vertebrae.

7. **What is skin traction?**

   Skin traction is used to control muscle spasms and to immobilize an area before surgery. Skin traction is accomplished by using weight to pull on traction tape or on a foam boot attached to the skin.

8. **What are clinical manifestations of fracture?**
   - Edema and swelling.
   - Pain and tenderness.
   - Deformity.
   - Echymosis.
   - Loss of function.
   - Crepitation.

9. List out the clinical manifestation of osteoporosis.

- Strain.
- Bump.
- Fall causes a hip, vertebral or wrist fracture.
- Collapsed vertebra may initially be manifested as back pain, loss of height, or spinal deformities.
- Limited ability to perform ADL

10. Define dislocation.

Dislocation is a severe injury of the ligamentation structures that surround a joint. Dislocation results in the complete displacement or separation of the articular surface of the joint.

11. What are risk factors for osteoarthritis?

- Increased age
- Obesity
- Previous joint damage
- Repetitive use
- Anatomic deformity
- Genetic susceptibility

12. What do you mean by osteomyelitis?

Osteomyelitis is an infection of the bone. The bone become infected because of extension of soft tissue infection, direct bone contamination from bone surgery and hematogenous spread from other sites of infection.

13. What is sprain?

Sprain is an injury to the ligaments and supporting muscle fibers that surround a joint. It is caused by a wrenching or twisting motion.

14. What is strain?

A strain or a pulled muscle is an injury to a musculoteunous unit caused by overuse, overstretching or excessive stress.

15. What is dislocation?

A dislocation of a joint is a condition in which articular surface of the bones forming the joint are no longer in anatomic fposition.

16. What is epicondylitis (Tennis elbow)?

Epicondylitis is a chronic, painful condition caused by excessive, repetitive extension, flexion, pronation and supination activities of the forearm.

17. What is fracture?

A fracture is a break in the continuity of bone and is defined according to its type and extent. Fracture is caused by direct blows, crushing forces, sudden twisting and extreme muscle contraction.

18. List down the types of fracture.

- Complete fracture
- Incomplete fracture
- Comminuted fracture
- Open fracture

19. What are classical manifestations of fracture?

- Pain is continuous and increase in severity until the bone fragment is immobilized.
- Loss of function.
- Displacement, angulations or rotation of the fragment on a fracture of the arm or leg cause a deformity.
- Shortening.
- Crepitus.
- Swelling and discoloration.

20. Explain Buck's extension traction.

Buck's extension traction is a skin traction to the lower leg. The pull is exerted one plane when partial or temporary immobilization is desired. It is used to immobilize fractures of the proximal femur before surgical fixation.

21. What are the nursing management of the patient with hip replacement?

- Preventing dislocation of the hip prosthesis.
- Monitoring wound drainage.
- Preventing infection.
- Promoting home and community based case.

22. What is the meaning of amputation?

Amputation is the removal of a body part usually an extremity. Amputation is used to release symptoms, to improve function and most importantly to save or improve the patient's quality of life.

23. Explain principles of traction.

- Traction must be continuous to be effective in reducing and immobilizing fractures.
- Skeletal traction is never interrupted.
- Weights are not removed unless intermittent traction is prescribed.

24. Define carpal tunnel syndrome.

Carpal tunnel syndrome is an entrapment neuropathy that occurs when the median nerve at the wrist is compressed by a thickened flexor tendon sheath, skeletal encroachment; edema or soft tissue mass. The syndrome is commonly caused by repetitive hand and wrist movements.

25. What are complications of fracture?

- **Shock:** Hypovolemic shock resulting from hemorrhage and from loss of intravascular volume into the interested space.
- **Fat embolism syndrome:** Afțer fracture of long bone or pelvic bones, multiple fracture fat embolisms may develop at the time of fracture, fat globules may diffuse into the vascular compartment because the marrow pressure is greater than the capillary pressure.

26. What is dystrophy?

It is a group of genetically transmitted disease characterized by progressive symmetric wasting of skeletal muscle without evidence of neurologic involvement. In all case of muscular dystrophy an insidious loss of strength occurs with increasing disability and deformity.

27. List out the clinical manifestation of intervertebral lumbar disc damage.

- Low back pain.
- Reduction pain that radiates down the buttock and below the knee.
- Reflexes may be depressed or absent.
- paresthesia or muscle weakness in the legs, feet.
- Multiple nerve root (cauda equina) compression may be manifested as bowel and bladder incontinence or impotence.

28. List types of ortho surgeries.

- **Synovectomy:** It is the removal of synovial membrane is used as a prophylactic measure and as a palliative treatment of rheumatoid arthritis.
- **Osteotomy:** It is performed by removing or adding a wedge or slice of bone to change ligament and to shift weight bearing, thereby correcting deformity and relieving pain.
- **Debridement:** it is the removal of degenerative debris such as loose bodies, osteophytes, joint debris and degenerated muscle from a joint.
- **Arthroplasty:** it is the reconstruction or replacement of joint.

29. Define Osteochondroma.

It is primary benign bone tumor the characterized by an overgrowth of cartilage and near the end of the bone at the growth plate. Osteochondroma can occur in any bone where cartilage assists in forming bone.

30. What are the preventive methods of low back pain?

- Maintain healthy weight.
- Do not sleep in a prone position.
- Avoid cigarette smoking and tobacco products.
- Obtain regular physical activity.
- Use proper body mechanism.
- Sleep one side with knees flexed.

31. List out the causes of neck pain.

- Poor posture.
- Strain or sprain.
- Degenerative disc disease.
- Spondylosis.
- Rheumatoid arthritis.
- Tumour.
- Osteoporosis.
- Osteomyelitis
- Meningitis.

32. What are the complications of rheumatoid arthritis?

Without treatment, joint destruction begins as early as the first year of the disease nodular myositis and muscle fiber degeneratiuon can lead to pain similar to that of vascular insufficiency cataract development and loss of vision can result from scleral muscles. Complication can also result from rheumatoid modules.

33. What are the criteria for rheumatoid arthritis?

- Morning stiffness that lasts.
- Swelling in three or more joints.
- Swelling in hand joints.
- Symmetric joint swelling.
- Rheumatoid nodules.

34. What is ankylosing spondylitis?

It is a chronic inflammatory disease that primarily affect the skeleton including the sacroiliac joints, intervertebral disc space and costovertebral articulation.

35. Define spondyloarthropathies.

It is group of interrelated multisystem inflammatory disorder that affect the spine, peripheral joint and articular structures.

36. Define traction.

It is the application of pulling force to an injured or diseased part of the body or an extremity while counter traction pulls in the opposite direction.

37. What is rheumatic disease?

Rheumatic disease are commonly called as arthritis but they are actually more than 100 different type of disorders that primarily affect skeletal muscles, bones, cartilage, ligaments, tenders and joints.

38. What are the common manifestations in rheumatic disease?

Pain is the most common symptoms other symptoms include joint swelling, limited movement, stiffness, weakness and fatigue.

39. What is arthrocentesis?

Arthrocentesis is a needle aspiration of synovial fluid may be performed not only to obtain a sample of synovial fluid for analysis but also to relieve pain caused by the pressure of increased fluid volume usually the knee or shoulder.

40. Explain purpose of traction?

- Prevent or release muscle spasm.
- Immobilize joint or part of the body.
- Reduce a fracture or dislocation.

- Treat a pathologic condition.
- Provide immobilization to prevent soft tissue damage.
- Expand a joint space during arthroscopic procedure.
- Reduce muscle spasm associated with low back pain.
- Expand a joint space before joint reconstruct.

41. What is cast?

A cast is a temporary circumferential immobilization device. Casting is a common treatment following closed reduction. It allows the patient to perform many normal activities of daily living while providing sufficient immobilization to ensure stability.

42. What are the types of cast?

Short arm cast: It is often used for treatment of stable wrist or metacarpal fracture. It is a circular last extending from the distal palmer area to the proximal forearm.

Long arm cast: It is commonly used for stable forearm or elbow fracture or unstable wrist fracture. It is similar to the short arm cast but extends to the proximal humerus, restricting motion in the wrist and elbow.

Body jacket cast: It is often used for immobilization and support for stable spine injuries of thoracic or lumbar spine.

Hip spine cast: It is used for treatment of femoral fracture the purpose of the hip spica cast is to immobilize the affected extremity and the treat securely.

43. Explain types of traction.

- **Skin traction:** It is used for short term treatment. Tape, boots or splints are applied directly to the skin to maintain alignment, assist in reduction.
- **Skeletal traction:** It is used for longer period. It is used to align injured bones and or to treat joint contracture and congenital hip dyplasica.

44. List out clinical manifestation of hip fracture.

- External rotation.
- Muscle spasm.
- Shortening of the affected extremity.
- Severe pain.
- Tenderness in the region of fracture site.

45. What is spinal stenosis?

It is narrowing of the vertebral canal or nerve root canals caused by an encroachment of bone on the space. The stenosis may be congenital or more typically it is through degenerative or traumatic changes to the spine.

46. Explain colles fracture.

It is the fracture of the distal radius and is one of the most common fracture in the adult. The styloid process of the ulna involved the injury usually occurs when the patient attempt to break a fall with an outstretched arm and hand.

47. What are clinical indications of amputation?

- Traumatic and thermal injuries
- Malignant tumors.
- Uncontrolled or wide spread infection of the extremity.
- Congenital disorder

48. What is CREST syndrome?

- C-Calcinosis
- R-Raynaud's phenomenon
- E-esophageal hardening
- S-Sclerodactyly
- T-Telangiectasis

49. What is polymyositis?

Polymyositis is one of a group of disease

termed idiopathic inflammatory myopathies. It is classified as autoimmune because auto antibodies are present.

50. What is meant by spondyloarthropathies?

They are another category of systemic inflammatory disorders of the skelton. They include ankylosing spondylitis, reactive arthritis, and psoiatic arthritis.

51. Define reiter's syndrome?

Reactive arthritis is otherwise called as reiter's syndrome, This disease process is called reactive because the arthritis occurs following an infection. It affects young adult males and is characterized primarily by urethritis, arthritis and conjunctivitis.

52. What is bursitis?

It is the inflammation of the bursa. Bursa is a closed sac such that are lined with synovial membrane and contain a small amount of synovial fluid. Bursitis results from repeated or excessive trauma or fracture, gout, rheumatoid arthritis or infection.

53. What is meant by repetitive strain injury?

It is the cumulative traumatic disorder resulting from prolonged, forceful awkward movement. It is also reported as repetitive trauma disorder. Repeated movements strain the tendon, ligaments and muscles causing tiny tears that become inflamed.

54. Define carpel tunnel syndrome.

It is a condition by compression of median nerve, which enters the hand though the narrow confines of the carpel tunnel, the carpel tunnel is formed by ligaments and bones.

55. What is mean by arthrocentesis?

Arthrocentesis or joint aspiration is usually performed for a synovial fluid analysis it may be used to instill medication for the patient with septic arthritis or to fluid from joints to relieve pain

56. What is arthroscopy?

A small fiberoptic tube called an anthroscope is used to directly examine the interior of joints, in this procedure anesthesia will give to patient.

57. What is compartment syndrome?

It is a condition in which elevated intra compartment pressure within a confined facial compartment compromise the neurovascular function of tissue within that space. Compartment syndrome cause capillary perfusion to be reduced below level necessary for tissue viability and is classified as acute, chronic or crush syndrome.

58. What is gout?

Gout is a heterogenous group of conditions related to a genetic defect of purine metablosim resulting in hyperuremia.

59. What are manifestations of gout syndrome?

Acute gouty arthritis, tophi, gouty nephropathy and uric acid urinary calculi.

60. What are the medications used to treat gout?

Colchicine - Lowers the deposition of uric acid and interferes with lacticacid production by leukocytes which results in a decrease in uric acid deposition and a reduction in phagocytosis, with abatement of the inflammatory response.

Probenacid - Uricosuric agent, inhibit renal reabsorption of urates and increases urinary excretion of uric acid prevents tophi formation.

61. What is meant by pannus?

Pannus is newly formed synovial tissue infilterated with inflammatory cells.

62. Mention medical management for rheu-

matoid arthritis

- Salicylate and NSAIDS
- Immuno suppressive agents
- Rest
- Exercise
- Range of motion
- Muscle strengthening exercise

63. What is polymyalgia rheumatica?

It is characterized by severe proximal muscle discomfort with mild joint swelling, severe aching in neck, shoulder and pelvic muscles. Immunoglobulin deposits in the walls of inflammed temporal arteries, also suggest an autoimmune process. An association with genetic marker HLA-DR4 suggests a familial predisposition.

Test Series XI

1. **What is apoptosis?**
   It is programmed cell death, it is the body's way of destroying unwanted cells such as cancer cells or cells that have natural death.
2. **What are three common modes of HIV transmission?**
   - Sexual transmission
   - Contact with blood and blood products
   - Prenatal transmission
3. **What is atopy?**
   Atopy refers to allergic reactions characterized by the action of IgE antibodies and a genetic predisposition to allergic reactions.
4. **List different types of immunoglobulin.**
   The body can produce five different types of Immunoglobulin. They are
   - IgG constitutes 75% of immunoglobulins
   - IgA constitutes 15% of immunoglobulins
   - IgM constitutes 10 of immunoglobulins
   - IgD constitutes 0.2%
   - IgE constitutes 0.004%
5. **Explain acute retroviral syndromes.**
   Fever, swollen lymph glands, sore throat, headache, malaise, nausea, muscle and joint pain, diarrhea, diffuse rash occur 1 to 3 weeks after initial infection and last for 1-2 weeks.
6. **What is the role of B cells?**
   The B cell or B lymphocyte is programmed to produce one specific antibody. On encountering a specific antigen, a B cell stimulates production of plasma cells, the site of antibody production, the result is the outpouring of antibodies for the purpose of destroying and removing the antigen.
7. **What is meant by primary immunodeficiencies?**
   They are rare diseases with genetic origins and are seen primarily in infants and young children. More than 95 immunodeficiencies of genetic origin have been identified so far.
8. **List primary immunodeficiency disorder.**
   - Hyperimmunoglobulinemia E syndrome
   - Sex-linked a gammaglobulinemia
   - Common variable immunodeficiency
   - Immunoglobulin A deficiency
   - Chronic mucocutaneous candidiasis
   - Wiskott-aldrich Syndrome
   - Sever combined immunodeficiency disease

- paroxysmal nocturnal hemoglobinuria

9. Write any 5 warning signs of primary immunedeficiencies?

- Eight or more new ear infections within a year
- Two or more serious sinus infection within a year
- Two or more months on antibiotics with little effect
- Two or more pneumonias within 1year
- Failure of an infant to gain weight or grow normally

10. What is agammaglobulinemia?

It is a disorder market by an almost complete lack of immunoglobulins or antibodies.

11. What is ataxia– telangiectasia?

It is a disorder market by an almost complete lack of immunoglobulins or antibodies.

12. What is SCID?

SCID is a phenotypic term that is used for a wide variety of congenital and hereditary immunologic defects that are characterized by early onset of infections, defects in both T cell and B cell systems.

13. Define Wiskott-Aldrich syndrome.

It is an immunodeficiency characterized by thrombocytopenia and the absence of T and B cells

14. What is Di George syndrome?

It is also called thymic hypoplasia, an example for primary T-cell immunodeficiency. This rare congenital disease results form the absence of several genes on chromosome 22.

15. Define the term immunity?

It is the resistance usually associated with the possession of antibodies for a specific disease. There are 2 types-Active & passive immunity.

16. What is the role of T cells and B cells?

T lymphoctes assist the B cells in producing antibodies. T cells secrete substances known as lymphokines that encourage cell growth, promote cell activation, direct the flow of cell activity, destroy target cells and stimulate the macrophagia.

17. What are the two different groups of antigens?

Complete protein antigens, such as animal dander pollen and horse serum stimulates complete humoral response.

18. List down primary chemical mediators of hypersensitivity.

- Histamine
- Eosinophil chemotactic factor of anaphylaxis
- Platelet-activating factor
- Prostaglandins

19. List down secondary chemical mediators of hypersensitivity.

Leukotriens, bradykinin, serotonin, heparin.

20. What are the four different types of hypersensitivity reactions?

- Type I anaphylactic hypersentivity
- Cytotoxic hypersensitivity type II
- Immune complex hypersensitivity type III
- Delayed type hypersensitivity type IV

21. Mention the pharmacological management in rheumatic disease.

- Salicylates
- NSAIDS
- Immunosuppressive (methotrexate, cyclophosphamide, cyclosporine
- Coritcosteriods (Prednisolone, Hydrocortosone)
- Topical analgesic (Capsaicin)

22. List down the surgical management of rheumatid arthritis.

- Synovectomy – Excision of synovial membrane
- Tenorrhaphy – Suturing the tendon
- Arthodesis-Surgical fusion of the joint
- Arthroplasty-Surgical repair and replacement of the joint

23. What is SLE?

Systemic lupus erythematosis is a result of disturbed immune regulation that causes an exaggerated production of auto antibodies. This immunoregulatory disturbance is brought about by some combination of genetic hormonal and environmental factors.

24. Mention one the drugs that induce SLE?

Hydralazine, procainaminde, isoniazid, chlorpromazine and some antiseizure medications.

25. What are the common skin manifestations in SLE?

Papulosquamous or annular polycyclic lesions and discoid lupus erythematosus which is a chronic rash that has erythematous papules or plaques and sealing and can cause scarring and pigmentation changes. Common lesions are butterfly shaped rash across the bridge of the nose and cheeks.

26. What are the biological theories?

- Crosslink theory.
- Free radical theory.
- Immunologic theory.
- Wear and tear theory.

27. What are the complications of rheumatoid arthritis?

Without treatment, joint destruction begins as early as the first year of the disease. Nodular myositis and muscle fiber degeneration can lead to pain similar to that of vascular insufficiency, cataract development and loss of vision can result from scleral muscles. Complication can also result from rheumatoid modules.

28. What are the criteria for rheumatoid arthritis?

- Morning stiffness that lasts.
- Swelling in three or more joints.
- Swelling in hand joints.
- Symmetric joint swelling.
- Rheumatoid nodules.

29. Explain the pharmacologic management of SLE.

- NSAIDs For minor manifestation
- Oral or intravenous corticosteroids
- Anti malarial medications
- immunosuppressive agents

Test Series XII

1. **What do you mean by communicable disease?**
An illness due to a specific infectious agent (or) toxic products which arises through transmission of that agent (or) its products from a reservoir to a susceptible host either directly or indirectly through vector an intermediate plant (or) animal host or the inanimate environment.
2. **What is the causative organism for chickenpox & its incubation period?**
Varicella zoster (V-Z) virus. Its incubation period is 14-16 days.
3. **Define scarlet fever.**
It is a contagious disease. Its occurrence is most common in temperature zones. Rarely seen among 5-6 years age group. Streptococcus pyogenes is the causative organism.
4. **List down 4 nursing diagnosis for meningococcal meningitis.**
   - Ineffective cerebral tissue perfusion related to neuromuscular dysfunction as evidenced by headache.
   - Impaired thermoregulation related to inflammatory process.
   - Activity intolerance related to stiffness of neck, neuromuscular dysfunction & fatigue.
   - Risk for injury related to seizure activity.
5. **What is the clinical spectrum for poliomyelitis?**
Inapparent infection 96%, abrupt onset with fever, which lasts for 1-6 days (104°F), malaise, lassitude, chills, severe headache, backache, pain in limb, vomiting, diarrhea, abdominal pain.
6. **Define carriers.**
An infected person (or) animal that harbors a specific infectious agent in the absence of clinical disease & serves as a potential source of infection for man.
7. **List down the main clinical features of chickenpox.**
Moderate fever, pain in the back, shivering & malaise, rashes. It develops through the stages of macule, papule, vesicle, scab & pleomorphism.
8. **Explain the management of scarlet fever?**
   - Suspected cases noted and reported to the health authorities
   - Health education
   - Milk must be pasteurized or boiled properly before using it
   - Infected persons should not handle milk or food to prevent contamination.
   - Sulphonamides 0.5-1gm/day, 2 lakh to 2 lakh 50 thousand unit's penicillin on empty stomach twice a day should

be given.

9. What is ARI?

Acute respiratory infection is caused by inflammation of respiratory tract anywhere from nose to alveoli with wide range of combination of symptoms & signs.

10. What are the types of vaccines used in poliomyelitis?

Inactivated (salk) polio vaccine, oral (sabin) polio vaccine.

11. What is hepatitis B immunoglobin?

For immediate protection, it is used for those exposed to HBsAg positive blood. It is given in 6 hours (ie) 0.05-0.07ml/kg body weight.

12. Define disinfection.

Killing of infectious agent by using chemical externally.

13. What do you mean by endemic?

The constant pressure of the disease within a given geographical area.

14. Define epidemic?

The occurrence or outbreak of an infectious disease in a community in excess of normal expectancy.

15. Define incubation period.

The time (or) interval between exposure to an infectious agent (or) person & appearance.

16. Define isolation.

The separation of infected person from normal persons, so as to avoid spread of infection for the period of communicability.

17. What is susceptibility?

A person not possessing sufficient resistance against a particular pathogenic agent to prevent contracting the infection.

18. Mention the diagnostic criteria for AIDS.

- CD4+T cells count drops below 200 cells/uL
- Development of anyone of the opportunistic infections
- Development of one of the opportunistic cancers.
- Wasting syndrome occurs
- Dementia develops

19. What are the common opportunistic cancers in HIV infection?

- Invasive cervical cancer
- Kaposis sarcoma
- Burkitt's lymphoma
- Immunoblastic lymphoma
- Primary lymphoma of brain

20. What are the common lab tests for diagnosing HIV?

- ELIZA (Enzyme linked immunosorbent assay)
- Western blot
- Viral load
- CD/CD 8 ratio

21. Mention classification of anti retroviral agents.

- Nucleoside reverse transcriptase inhibitors
- Non nucleoside reverse transcriptase inhibitors
- Protease Inhibitors
- Fusion Inhibitors

22. List down nucleoside reverse transcriptase inhibitors.

Zidovudine, didanosine, zalcitabine, staridome, lamirudine, abacavir, combivir

23. List down protease inhibitors and in HIV infection.

Sagunivir, indinavir, ritnavir, nelfinavir, amprenavir

24. Define surveillance of disease?

It is the continuing scrutiny of all aspects of occurrence & spread of a disease that are pertinent to effective control.

25. What is the prophylactic intervention for PCP?

Trimethoprim drugs-sulfamethoxazole or dapsone with otrunetganube and folinic acid, aerosolized pentamidine, atoraguone.

26. What is the prophylaxis for MAC?

Mycobacterium avium complex (MAC) Clavitaromycin or azirthromycin, rifabutin Prophylaxis discontinued if immuno reconstruction evident.

27. What is mode of transmission for measles?

Directly from person to person mainly by droplet infection & droplet nuclei from 4 days before onset of rash until 5 days thereafter.

28. List down the stages of clinical features in measles.

- Prodromal stage
- Eruptive phase,
- Post measles phase.

29. Write down the complications of measles.

Mainly neurological complications they are febrile convulsions, encephalitis, subactue sclerosing panencephalitis characterized by mental deterioration leading to paralysis, probably due to persistence of the virus in the brain.

30. How can measles be prevented?

- Achieving an immunization rate of over 95%
- Ongoing immunization against measles through successive generations of children.
- Immunisation: Before the age of 9 months
- S/c 0.5ml, vaccine stored at 4-8 degree, mild illness (fever or rash) 5-10 days after immunization.

31. Define diphtheria.

It is an acute infectious disease caused by toxigenic strains of corynebacterium diphtheriae.

32. What is the mode of transmission of diphtheria?

The disease spreads mainly by droplet infection. It can be transmitted directly to susceptible persons from infected cutaneous lesions.

33. What is Schick test?

It is an intradermal test. The test is carried out by injecting intradermal into the skin of forearm 0.2ml of schick toxin,"control" the same amount of toxin which has been inactivated by heat.

34. What are the clinical manifestations of diphtheria?

Pharyngo tonsillar, laryngotracheal, nasal mild erythema on the throat, localized or a membrane early stage whitish-thick blue-white to grey black adherent, bull necked appearance.

35. What is another name for whooping cough?

The another name of whooping cough is called as pertussis,

36. What is the incubation period for whooping cough?

Incubation is 7 to14 days.

37. List complications of whooping cough?

- Haemorrhage (skin, ear, gums)
- Bronchitis
- Pulmonary collapse
- Bronchopneumonia
- Lung fibrosis
- Cerebral haemorrhage
- Encephalitis

- Convulsions
- Paralysis of different parts of body
- Spasm of glottis
- Hernia
- Ulcer of frenulum

38. What are the prophylaxis for diphtheria?

Combined (or) mixed vaccine - DPT, DT, Dt (diphtheria tetanus, adult type), single vaccine, antisera.

39. Define meningococcal meningitis?

Meningococcal meningitis/ cerebrospinal fever are an acute communicable disease caused by neisseria meningitidis.

40. What is the mantoux test?

The mantoux test is carried out by injecting intradermally on the flex or surface of the forearm TU - 0.1 ml. The induration in the hand is measured to find out the disease. More than 10 mm then the case is positive & less than 6 mm the case is negative.

41. What are factors responsible for tuberculosis?

Age, sex, hereditary, nutrition, immunity

42. Is there a drug to treat tuberculosis? Explain with reason?

- **Bactericidal drugs:** Rifampicin 10-12mg/kg body weight), INH 4-5mg/kg of bodyweight streptomycin 0.75-1gm
- **Bacteriostatic drugs:** Ethambutol 15mg/kg body weight given in 2-3doses, thioacetazone 2mg/kg bodyweight

43. What is DOTS?

Directly Observed Treatment Short Course. It has 2 phases: Active phase, the patient takes the medicine in front of the health worker or trained person. Continuation phase is checked by return of empty multiblister combi pack when the patient comes to collect next medicine for next week.

44. What is the vaccine required for TB?

BCG vaccines live 0.05ml for the newborn I/D using tuberculin syringe.

45. When was TB programme started and revised?

In 1962 is started and revised in he year 1992

46. What is poliomyelitis?

It is the acute viral infection caused by a RNA virus. It is primarily an infection of the human alimentary tract but the virus may infect the CNS.

47. What is the mode of transmission and incubation period for poliomyelitis?

Faecal oral route, droplet infection. Incubation period is 7-14 days.

48. What are the contraindications for administering OPV?

Acute infectious disease, fever, diarrhea, dysentery, leukemia and those receiving corticosteroids.

49. List down two strategies for polio eradication in India?

- Conduct pulse polio immunization days every for 3-4 years until it is eradicated
- Sustain high levels of routine immunization coverage.

50. What is mopping?

These activities are done in the last stage of eradication programme, it involves door to door immunization in high risk districts.

51. When was pulse polio immunisation started? Define the term.

Started in the year 1995. The vaccine is given all over in the same day that is why it is said to be Pulse Polio Immunisation.

52. What are different types of hepatitis?

Hepatitis A, B, C, D, E, G.

53. What are 3 distinct antigens of hepatitis B virus?

A surface antigen HBsAg, a core antigen HBcAg, a "e" antigen HBeAg.

Test Series XIII

1. **Define ambulatory surgery.**
   It may include outpatient surgery that does not require an overnight hospital stay or short stay, with admission to an inpatient hospital setting for less than 24 hours.
2. **What are the various categories of surgery based on urgency?**
   a) Emergent b) Urgent c) Required
   d) Elective e) Optional
3. **Define circulating nurse?**
   Registered nurse who coordinates and documents patient care in the operating room.
4. **What are the two possible nursing diagnosis for intraoperative period.**
   - Anxiety related to expressed concerns.
   - Disturbed sensory perception related to general anesthesia or sedation.
5. **Define intraoperative phase.**
   It is the period of time from when the patient is transferred to the operating room table to when he or she is admitted to the post anesthesia care unit (PACU)
6. **Mention the aspects of perioperative patient focused model.**
   Physiological responses, behavioural responses, health system, safety.
7. **What are the activities of a scrub nurse?**
   Performing a surgical hand rub, setting up the sterile tables, preparing sutures, ligatures and special equipment, assisting the surgeon and surgical assistants and Sending the tissue specimens
8. **What are the two phases of post anesthesia care unit?**
   Phase 1: Used during the immediate recovery phase
   Phase 2: Less frequent observation and less nursing care required
9. **Define perioperative phase.**
   It is the period of time that constitutes the surgical experience; includes the preoperative, intraoperative and postoperative phases of nursing care.
10. **Define postoperative phase.**
    It is the period of time that begins with the admission of the patient to the PACU (Post Anesthesia Care Unit) and ends after a follow up evaluation in the clinical setting or home.
11. **Define preoperative phase.**
    It is the period of time from when the decision for surgical intervention is made to when the patient is transferred to the operating room table.
12. **What is PAT?**
    PAT means Pre Admission Testing. It is the

diagnostic testing performed before admission to the hospital.

13. What are the phases of perioperative nursing?

- Preoperative
- Intraoperative
- Postoperative

14. What is informed consent?

It is the patient's autonomous decision about whether to undergo a surgical procedure; based on the nature of the condition, the treatment options and the risks and benefits involved.

15. What are the components of informed consent?

- Explanation of procedure and its risks.
- Description of benefits and alternatives
- An offer to answer a questions about procedure
- Instructions that the patient may withdraw consent.

16. When do we need to take consent?

Informed consent is necessary in the following circumstances.

- Invasive procedures such as surgical incision, a biopsy, cystoscopy, a paracenthesis
- Procedures requiring sedation and/or anesthesia
- A non surgical procedure, such as arteriography, that carries more than slight risk to the patient
- Procedures involving radiation.

17. Enumerate the preoperative instructions to be given to prevent postoperative complications.

- Diaphragmatic breathing
- Coughing
- Leg Exercises
- Turning to the side
- Getting out of bed

18. Define diaphragmatic breathing.

Diaphragmatic breathing refers to the flattening of the dome of the diaphragm during inspiration with resultant enlargement of the upper abdomen as air rushes enduring expiration, the abdominal muscles contract.

19. Give examples for cognitive coping strategies?

Imagery
Distraction
Optimistic self recitation

20. List pre operative psycho social intervention.

- Reducing pre operative anxiety
- Decreasing fear
- Respecting cultural, spiritual and religious beliefs

21. What are the general pre operative interventions?

- Managing nutrition and fluids
- Preparing the bowel for surgery
- Preparing the skin
- Administering preanesthetic medications
- Maintaining the pre operative record
- Transporting the patient to presurgical area
- Attending to family needs

22. List down two nursing diagnosis for pre operative phase.

- Anxiety related to outcome of surgery
- Fear related to perceived threat of surgical procedure

23. Define anesthesia.

It is defined as a state of narcosis, analgesia, relaxation and loss of reflexes.

24. Define surgical asepsis.

Absence of micro organisms in the surgical environment to reduce the risk of infection

25. List down some effects of anesthesia.
- Cardiac dysrhythmias
- Myocardial depression
- Malignant hyperthermia
- Hypotension

26. What are the health hazards associated with surgical environment?
- Laser risks
- Exposure to blood and body fluids
- Latex allergy

27. What are the four levels of sedation and anesthesia?

Minimal, moderate, deep sedation and anesthesia

28. What are the four stages of general anesthesia?
- Stage 1 Beginning anesthesia
- Stage 2 Excitement
- Stage 3 Surgical anesthesia
- Stage 4 Medullary depression

29. Mention the various methods of anesthesia administration.
- Inhalation • Intravenous • Regional
- Conduction blocks and anesthesia
- Local filtration anesthesia

30. Name local anesthetic agents.
- Lidocaine • Etidocaine
- Procaine • Tetracaine

31. Mention the potential intra operative complications.
- Nausea and vomiting
- Anaphylaxis
- Hypoxia and other respiratory complications
- Hypothermia

32. Define malignant hypothermia.

It is an inherited muscle disorder chemically induced by anesthetic agents.

33. What are the classic signs of shock?

Pallor, cool, moist skin, rapid breathing, cyanosis of the lips, gums and tongue, rapid weak and thready pulse, decreasing pulse pressure, low B.P and concentrated urine.

34. What are the two types of hemorrhage?

Evident and concealed.

35. What are the complications of post operative period?

Atelectasis, pneumonia, pulmonary embolism, aspiration, shock, thrombophlebitis, infection, dehiscence.

36. Write two possible nursing diagnoses for post operative period.
- Acute pain related to surgical incision
- Decreased cardiac output related to shock or hemorrhage

37. Name the three mechanisms of wound healing.
- First • Second • Third intention healing

38. What are the phases of wound healing?
- Inflammatory
- Proliferative
- Maturation

39. List factors affecting wound healing.
- Age
- Nutritional deficits
- Medications
- Systemic disorders
- Immune depressed state

40. List nursing interventions during post operative period.
- Preventing respiratory complications
- Promoting wound healing
- Promoting bowel function
- Relieving pain
- Promoting cardiac output
- Encouraging activity
- Maintaining normal body temperature

PATHOLOGY

INTRODUCTION

Pathology is the scientific study of disease. It mainly focuses on the study of the structural a-nd functional changes in cells, tissues and organs of the body. Pathology is a vital component of medical education. Pathology knowledge is fundamental to modern medical practice and health care.

Various techniques used to study pathology includes surgical pathology, cyto-pathology and hematology. The disease is studied under the following aspects: etiology, pathogenesis, morphologic changes, clinical manifestations, prognosis and complications.

Inflammation

Inflammation is a complex local response of the living vascularized tissues to injury. It mainly consists of responses of blood vessels and leukocytosis.

Cardinal signs of inflammation are rubor, tumor, colar, dolor and loss of function.

Wound healing is a process of replacement of dead tissues by living tissue. Healing may be by regeneration or by repair.

Electrolytes are the chemicals or salts that have an electric changes. Electrolytes are ions either positively or negatively charged.

Neoplasia

Neoplasia means new growth. The new growth formed is known as neoplasm. Oncology is the study of tumors or neoplasms. Tumors can be classified in to benign and malignant.

Clinical pathology

Anticoagulants are used to prevent blood from clotting. Commonly used anti-coagulants is calcium chelating agents which includes heparin, EDTA.

Hemoglobin is estimated by calorimetric methods, physical methods, chemical methods, gasometric method etc.

Hemogram includes RBS, total and differential leucocyte count, platelet count, PCV, ESR and peripheral smear. The hemocytometer is an instrument used for counting blood cells. It includes REC pipette, WBC pipette and improved neubaucer counting chamber.

Blood chemistry: The basic blood tests are done to assess a wide range of conditions and the functions of organs. The blood substances measured in the basic tests varies depending on the clinical features and the provisional diagnosis. The common tests include: measurement of electrolytes, blood urea nitrogen, creatinine, blood glucose etc.

Bone marrow examination is essentially done to rule out a hematologic conditions.

CSF analysis is a diagnostic importance in CNS conditions with CSF involvement.

Body fluids examinations: The commonly examined body fluids in the laboratory include pleural, pericardial, peritoneal and synovial fluid.

References

1. Nayak R, Rai S, Gupta A (2013). **Textbook of Pathology and Genetics for Nurses.** 1st ed. Jaypee
2. Mohan H (2008). **Textbook of Pathology.** 4th ed. Jaypee.
3. Tanushweta. **Review of Pathology.** 2nd ed. Jaypee.

Test Series

1. **Define pathology.**
   Pathology is the scientific study of diseases or the study of structural and functional changes in disease.
2. **Define etiology.**
   Diseases are expression of 'discomfort' due to structural and functional abnormalities. These abnormalities can be caused by various agents like bacteria, virus, heat, radiation etc., are collectively called etiology, The study of disease causing agent.
3. **Define pathogenesis.**
   It is the study of disease progression or evolution.
4. **Define morphology.**
   It is the study of structural changes in disease- Gross and microscopic.
5. **Define clinical significance.**
   It is the study of how clinical features are related to various changes. The science of pathology helps us to reach a diagnosis in a disease state.
6. **What is Ghon complex?**
   Ghon focus along with the lymph node involvement is called Ghon complex.
7. **What are complications of bronchiectasis?**
   - **Pulmonary**

     Bronchopneumonia

     Abscess

     Gangrene
   - **Pleural**

     Dry Pleurisy

     Empyema

     Pyo-Pneumothorax
   - Pericarditis
   - Septicaemia and pyaemia

   5. Cerebral abscess
8. **Name the types of pneumonia.**
   On the basis of etiology:
   - Bacterial Pneumonia
   - Metastatic Pneumonia
   - Viral Pneumonia
   - Rickettsial Pneumonia
   - Protozoal Pneumonia
   - Aspiration Pneumonia

   On the basis of mode of spread:

   1. Acute pneumonia
   - Lobar pneumonia
   - Broncho pneumonia
   - Embolic Pneumonia

   2. Chronic interstitial pneumonia
9. **What are stages of lesions in pneumonia?**
   - Congestion
   - Red hepatization

- Grey hepatization
- Resolution

10. What are the substance causing pneumoconiosis?

- Silica (Silicosis)
- Coal dust
- Asbestos dust (Asbestosis)
- Graphite (Graphite fibrosis)
- Hayer corn dust (Farmer's Lung)

11. What is mendelson's syndrome?

It is a type of inhalation group of lung abscesses caused by aspiration of stomach contents into the lungs during obstetrical anesthesia.

Two factors play a part in its protection.

- Gastric Retention
- Laryngeal Paralysis

12. Name the 4 forms of emphysema.

- Chronic obstructive emphysema
- Complementary emphysema
- Senile atrophic emphysema
- Interstitial emphysema

13. What are the 3 historical types of the malignant tumors of the lung?

- Epidermoid (Squamous cell carcinoma)
- Anaplastic (Small cell, reserve cell carcinoma)
- Adenocarcinoma

14. Define achalasia and write its abnormalities.

Achalasia means failure to relax. It is characterized by 3 major abnormalities.

- Aperistalsis
- Partial or incomplete relaxation of the LES (Lower esophageal sphincter) with swallowing
- Increase resting tone of LES

15. What are the types of gastritis?

1. Acute gastritis

- Catarrhal gastritis
- Membranous gastritis
- Phelgmonous gastritis

2. **Chronic gastritis**

- Superficial Gastritis
- Atrophic Gastritis
- Gastric Atrophy

16. What is the solution used for preservation of blood?

Acid citrate dextrose (ACD)

17. Write about specimen collection for CSF analysis?

CSF is collected by lumbar puncture needle. This needle measures 10-12 cm in length. It consists of a needle and a stick. The client is flexed in lateral position with knees drawn up. The third lumbar space is cleaned with spirit and needle. This needle is passed through supraspinous ligaments. The stick is withdrawn and CSF collected in sterile container.

18. Explain about the CSF on gross examination.

The CSF is examined for colour, appearance and formation of coagula. Normal CSF is colour less and clear. Yellow colour or xanthochromia is seen in subarachnoid bleed or severely jaundiced patient. Pink to red colour indicates the presence of blood. Turbid appearance is seen in the presence of numerous bacteria and cells. Coagula or clot formation standing resembles cobweb in tuberculosis meningitis.

19. What are the types of urine samples?

- Early morning sample – PH
- **Random specimen** – Microscopic examination
- **Second voided sample** – Urine sugar
- **Timed sample** – 24 hours urine sample

20. What is the routine examination of urine?

- Physical Examination
- Chemical Examination

21. What is diagnosis?

It is the formal name(s) used to describe patient's disease. It is the process of identifying a disease based on the patient's symptom's, the doctor's findings and the results of investigation and laboratory tests.

22. Why do we need to make a diagnosis?

It is a system of classification that supports necessary names, the findings and the result of investigations and laboratory tests. It is the means to ascertain the defining characteristics of a disease in the individual patient.

23. List down the subdivisions of pathology.

- Histopathology
- Cytopathology
- Hematology
- Immunology
- Chemical Pathology
- Genetics
- Forensic
- Pathology

24. Define general pathology.

It is the study of common changes in all tissues or the disease process as for example inflammation, cancer, ageing etc…

25. Define systemic pathology.

It is the study of specific changes in organs or the disease itself as for e.g.: Goiter, pneumonia, breast cancer etc.

26. What are typhoid intestine and its stages?

In the intestine, typhoid affects mainly the payer's patches and solitary follicles on the lower part of ileum. The various stages are:

- Acute inflammatory swelling of lymphoid tissue
- Necrosis
- Separation of dead tissue with formation of ulcer
- Process of healing

27. Name different types of cirrhosis of liver.

On the bass of pathological features, it can be classified as

- Portal cirrhosis
- Post necrotic cirrhosis
- Biliary cirrhosis
- Cardiac cirrhosis

28. Write about the characteristic lesion of chronic cholecystitis.

The characteristic lesion is accumulation of sub serous fat. The wall of gall bladder becomes thickened and fibrosed. There is a cavity filled with clear and colorless watery fluid secreted by lining epithelial cells. The condition is termed as mucocele of gall bladder.

29. What are the conditions for development of lung abscess?

- As a complication of necrotising pneumonia
- Aspiration of infective material from the GI tract or upper respiratory tract.
- Bronchial obstruction by tumor
- As a result of septic lung emboli.

30. What are the etiological factors of carcinoma endometrium?

- Obesity
- Diabetes
- Hypertension
- Consumption of exogenous estrogen
- Estrogen producing tumor

31. What is ectopic gestation?

Ectopic gestation is a form of extra uterine pregnancy. Here the implantation occurs outside the uterus. The sites where ectopic gestation can occur are the ovary, the fallopian tubes and the abdominal cavity.

32. What is fibroadenoma?

The most common benign tumor of the breast is fibroadenoma. This tumor is seen in young women. They present with solitary, discrete and mobile mass in the breast.

33. What is meningioma?

Meningioma is tumors that arise from the meninges which form the membranes covering the brain and spinal cord. They are usually capsulated, slow in growing and benign.

34. What is glioma?

Glioma's are neoplasm of supporting glial cells. Cerebral astrocytoma is the commonest type of glioma and occurs more in adult males. They are diffuse with no border as they infiltrate the surrounding time.

35. What are types of glioma?

- Ependymomas - Ependymal cells.
- Astrocytoma - Astrocytes
- Oligodendroma - Oligodendrocytes.

36. Mention the contraindication for bone marrow aspiration.

Congenital hemorrhagic disorder, hemophilia

37. What are the findings in microscopic examination for normal CSF?

Normal CSF does not contain RBC. WBC ranges from 0.8/microlit. This includes only lymphocytes.

- Cell count done in counting chamber.
- Differential count is done on Lieshman stained smear.

38. Describe the purpose of microbiological examination of CSF.

This help in finding out the specific etiological agents in cases of meningitis. These include gram stain, AFB stain, and CSF culture.

39. What are the colours of urine in various conditions?

- Normal urine - Amber colour
- Polyuria - Colourless
- Oliguria - Dark yellow orange
- Hemoglobinuria - Smoky colour or cola colour
- Jaundice - Yellow
- Alkaptonuria - Urine turns dark on standing

40. What are the causes of proteinuria?

- Seen in muscular exertion
- Hay fever
- Heavy metal poisoning
- Renal disease like nephrotic syndrome and acute glo-merular nephritis

41. Define amyloidosis.

It is a disease characterized by extracellular deposition in connective tissue of carbohydrate-protein material, amyloid.

42. What is cachexia?

It means body wasting and anemia usually associated with a neoplasm or chronic disease.

43. Mention classification of cachexia.

- Developmental— Genetic, congenital
- Inflammatory— Trauma, infections, immune diseases etc…
- Neoplastic— Tumors and cancers
- Degenerative— Ageing

44. What are the techniques used in diagnostic pathology?

- Gross pathology light microscopy
- Immuno histochemistry
- Electron microscopy
- Molecular pathology

45. Define a normal cell.

- The human cells are composed of the same basic components. It includes: Nucleus
- Cytoplasm
- Cell membrane

46. Define lymphedema.

It is due to obstruction of lymphatics causes excess of lymphatic fluid.

47. Define shock.

It is a state of hypo perfusion with blood.

48. What is acid fast bacillus?

Mycobacterium tuberculosis is a rod shaped bacterium with a waxy capsule. It is stained with Zeihl-Neelson technique. The bacterium takes a pink colour with this technique.

49. What is Langhan's giant cell?

Mycobacterium elicits the formation of granulomas. It does not attract the neutrophils at the site of infection. The granulomas are composed of lymphocytes and macrophages. The stimulated macrophages transform into epitheloid cells which often fuse to form multinucleated giant cells. These giant cells are also called Langhan's giant cells.

50. What is Ghon focus?

The primary infection in a person who has not been exposed to the organism previously results in the formation of a localized lung lesion. This is called as Ghon focus.

51. Define lung abscess.

Lung abscess is a localized suppurative destructive lesion which develops in the lung parenchyma.

52. Define pneumonia.

Pneumonia is defined as an infection in the lung. When the inflammation is mainly intra alveolar, it is called as alveolar pneumonia. If the inflammation predominantly involves the alveolar septa, it is called interstitial pneumonia.

53. Define bronchiectasis.

Bronchiectasis is a permanent dilatation of the bronchi and bronchioles caused by destruction of its elastic tissue and muscles.

54. What is bronchial asthma?

It is characterized by increased responsiveness of the bronchial tree to a variety of stimuli. The patients presents with recurrent wheezing episodes, breathlessness, tightness of chest and cough.

55. Define chronic bronchitis.

Excessive production of tracheobronchial mucus causing cough and expectoration for at least 3 consecutive months during 2 consecutive years.

56. What is heparin?

Heparin is an acidic substance normally present in the body in small amounts. It is used in the concentration of 0.1-0.2mg/ml of blood. It is used in osmotic fragility test and for electrolytic estimation in biochemistry.

57. What are the test included in the examination of CSF?

The CSF examination should be done within half-an hour of collection. Delay causes cell degradation as well as reduction in the glucose levels. Routine examination is done as follows:

- Gross/physical examination
- Microscopic examination
- Chemical examination

58. What are the abnormalities found on microscopic examination of CSF sample?

- An increase in the neutrophils is seen in bacterial meningitis, encephalitis, cerebral abscess and subdural empyema.
- An increase in the lymphocytes is seen in viral and tubercular meningitis and degenerative disorders.
- An increase in the eosinophil's is seen in parasitic infection and fungal infection.

59. What are the important inorganic constituents of urine?

Chloride, phosphorous, sulphur, sodium and potassium, urea, creatinine, uric acid and ammonia.

60. What is Helle's test?

2ml of con. nitric acid is taken in a test tube

with a pipette, urine run along the side of the test tube. Albumin gives a white ring at the junction.

61. Define hypertrophy.

Hypertrophy is increase in the size of the tissue or organ resulting from enlargement of individual cell.

62. Define hyperplasia.

Hyperplasia is an increase in the size of tissue or organ resulting from an increase in the number of cells.

63. What is atrophy?

Atrophy is the decrease in the size of the tissue or organ resulting from a decrease in the size of the cell.

64. List out the types of necrosis.

- Coagulative Necrosis
- Liquefactive Necrosi
- Caseous Necrosis
- Fat Necrosis

65. Define gangrene.

Gangrene is defined as "massive necrosis" with superadded putrefaction.

66. What are blue bloaters?

The patient with chronic bronchitis present with prominent cough with sputum. In severe cases, hyper apnea and hypoxemia causes cyanosis. Therefore these patients are described as blue bloaters.

67. Define emphysema.

It is a chronic obstructive airway disease characterized by permanent enlargement of airspace distal to terminal bronchioles.

68. Classify emphysema.

Emphysema classified into 4 forms:

- Centrilobular
- Panlobular
- Paraseptal
- Irregular

69. What is pleural effusion?

Accumulation of fluid in the pleural cavity is called pleural effusion. This is also called as hydrothorax.

70. What is atherosclerosis?

It is a systemic disease affecting the arteries. It is characterized by the formation of intimal lesions called atheroma which produce into the lumen of the artery.

71. Mention sites affected by atherosclerosis.

The common sites are coronary arteries, the arteries supplying the brain, the aorta and the arteries supplying the extremities.

72. What are complications of atherosclerosis?

- Rupture and ulceration of the plaque.
- Haemmorhage into the plaque.
- Atheroembolism
- Development of aneurysm.

73. What is pericardial effusion?

The pericardial sac contains around 30-50ml of fluid. It is a clear, straw coloured, serous fluid. Various conditions result in accumulation of more fluid in this cavity.

74. What is RHD?

Rheumatic fever is an acute, systemic, immunologically mediated disease which occurs a few weeks after an infection with group a beta hemolytic streptococcal pharyngitis.

75. Write about aschoff's body.

It is the lesion in the myocardium. It is made up of central degenerating hyper eosinophilic material infiltrated by lymphocytes, plasma cells and activated macrophages called aschoff's bodies.

76. What is hemocytometer?

It is an instrument used for counting blood cells. It consists of a counting chamber and 2 pipettes.

77. What is semen analysis?
Semen analysis is a technique to examine the semen which is done to investigate the cause of infertility.

78. Explain the purpose of semen analysis.
Semen analysis is done to investigate the cause of infertility. It account for 40%of cases of infertility. This test provides an important information about the quality and quantity of semen.

79. Write the composition of normal urine.
Water constitutes 95% of urine 2% urea 3% of organic and inorganic substances.

80. Write the diagnostic purposes of feces examination.
Stool sample is done to evaluate colorectal carcinoma, malabsorption, diarrheal disease and parasitic infestation.

81. Define cancer cell.
It is a group of neoplastic disease in which there is a transformation of normal cells into malignant cells. The cells proliferate in an abnormal way resulting in a malignant cellular tumor.

82. What are the causes of gangrene?
- Severance of an artery
- Rapid occlusion of an artery by compression from outside
- Spasm of the arterial wall
- Occlusion of the artery by a thrombus or an embolus.

83. Write about 'gas gangrene'.
It is caused by the exotoxins produced by the pathologic clostridia organisms.' Here the sugars are fermented producing gases. The gangrenous area is friable, a change best seen in the bowel.

84. Define exudates.
The increased permeability of vessel wall permitting the movement of protein rich fluid as well as cells into the interstitium. This fluid is called as an exudate.

85. Define edema.
The increased plasma osmotic pressure of the interstitium resulting in an accumulation of fluid in extra vascular or extracellular space is called as edema.

86. What is the cause of infective endocarditis?
It is caused by bacteria, fungi and rarely by ricketssiae and chlamydiae

87. What are the complications of myocardial infarction?
- Myocardial Rupture
- Ventricular Aneurysm
- Mural Thrombus.

88. What is aneurysm?
It is a localized abnormal dilatation of the lumen of the blood vessel.

89. What are the types of aneurysm?
- Saccular Aneurysm
- Fusiform Aneurysm
- Dissecting Aneurysm

90. List out the common diseases of GI tract.
- Dental carries
- Infectious diseases like gastroenteritis
- Peptic ulcer and inflammatory bowel disease
- Neoplasms

91. Define ulcer.
It is defined as a breach in the mucosa. In the alimentary tract, an ulcer extends through the muscularis mucosa into the sub mucosa.

92. List causative factors of peptic ulcer.
- Helicobacter pylori infection
- Mucosal exposure to gastric acid and pepsin
- Other factors include consumption of aspirin and NSAIDs, cigarette smok-

ing, alcohol consumption and duodenal gastric reflex.

93. What are the complications of peptic ulcer?
- Bleeding
- Perforation of the wall of the stomach and duodenum
- Rare complication include obstruction and malignant transformation

94. Mention causes of oral cancer.
- Smoking
- Chronic alcoholism
- Repeated trauma by sharp tooth
- UV light exposure
- Syphilis

95. Write morphologic types of carcinoma of the stomach.
- Fungating type.
- Ulcerating type.
- Diffuse infilterating type.

96. Mention the methods of haemoglobin estimation.
- Calorimetric method based on color.
- Physical method based on specific gravity.
- Chemical method based on iron content of hemoglobin.
- Gasometric method on oxygen carrying capacity of hemoglobin.
- Normal hemoglobin range -13.2-16.2 gm/dl in males.
- 12-15.2 gm/dl in females.

97. Mention the normal sperm count and its abnormal findings.

Normal sperm count is 40-300 millions/ ml

Count less than 20 million/ml is called as oligospermia.

Absence of sperms is called azoospermia.

98. Write about the processing of gastric and duodenal examination.

After obtaining the sample the mesh is retracted into the Teflon sheath, removed from the patient extruded from the sheath again and fixed in to the glass slides or used in a preservative solution.

99. What is sulpho salicyclic acid test?

2.5 ml of urine is taken in a test tube and 0.5 ml of 20% aqueous solution of sulpho salicyclic acid is added. Turbidity indicates the presence of protein.

100. Classify the deposits found during urine microscopy.

Organic deposits include casts, red blood cells, WBC, epithelial cells, bacteria, yeasts, parasite and spermatozoan.

In organic deposits Consist of crystalline or amorphous materials.

101. What is metastasis?

It is a tumor implant discontinuous with the primary tumor

102. List out the steps involved in metastasis.
- Detachment of the tumor cells from each other
- Attachment of the matrix components
- Degradation of the extracellular matrix
- Migration of the tumor cells.

103. Mention the laboratory diagnosis of cancer.
- Histological and cytological method
- Immunocytochemistry
- Molecular diagnosis
- Flow cytometry

104. Write the pathways for spread of cancer.
- Direct seeding of the body cavities or surfaces.
- Lymphatic spread.
- Hematogenic spread.

105. What are the common DNA viruses causing cancer?
- Human papilloma virus

- Epstein Barr virus
- Hepatitis B virus
- Herpes virus

106. What is the meaning of jaundice.

Jaundice refers to the yellowish discoloration of skin and mucosa caused by elevated serum bilirubin levels. Jaundice become apparent only if the bilirubin level is more than 2mg/dl.

107. List out the rate of transmission of viral hepatitis.

- Hepatitis A-Fecal oral route
- Hepatitis B-Parenteral, sexual contact
- Hepatitis C-Fecal oral route
- Hepatitis D-Fecal oral route
- Hepatitis-Paraenteral route

108. What is liver abscess?

It is a circumscribed collection of pus in the substance of liver.

109. Classify liver abscess and its causes.

- Pyogenic abscess- Enterobacteriae
- Amoebic liver abscess- Entamoeba histolytica
- Fungal abscess- Candida albicans.

110. State the types of gall stones.

- Cholesterol Stones
- Pigment Stones

111. Write the treatment of cholelithiasis.

Surgical removal or lithotripsy with antispasmodic and analgesic drugs.

112. What is cholecystitis and enlist the types of cholecystitis?

It is the inflammation of the gall bladder. It is of three types:

- Acute Calculous Cholecystitis.
- Acute Non Calculous
- Chronic Cholecystitis.

113. Write about the clinical features of cholecystitis.

- Severe upper abdominal pain with radiation to the right shoulder
- Fever, nausea, leukocytosis and prostration are common

114. List the clinical features of nephrotic syndrome.

- Edema
- Hypertension
- Hematuria
- Proteinuria
- Hypoalbuminemia

115. What is 'Goodpasture's syndrome?

This is an autoimmune disease characterized by the formation of antibodies to the body's own basement membrane component.

116. What is the normal bleeding time?

1-9 minutes.

117. Explain the normal sperm morphology.

A normal sperm has a head with an acrosomal cap which measures 4 micron in length. The middle piece is 7 micron in length between which lies a neck. The middle piece is followed by the tail measuring 45-50 micron in length.

118. What are the findings in sperm chemical examination?

Protein estimation is done which helps to differentiate a transudate and exudates.

119. What is the purpose of faeces examination?

Useful in evaluation of colorectal carcinoma, malabsorption, diarrhoeal disease and parasitic infestation.

120. List down the methods of preparation of stool sample for microscopy.

- Saline preparation
- Iodine preparation
- Stool concentration method
- Sample sedimentation method
- Normal saline ether sedimentation

method.

121. Define carcinogenesis.

It is the process by which a normal cell transforms into a malignant cell. It occurs in three ways:

Physical
Chemical
Viral.

122. What is chronic inflammation?

It is an inflammation for prolonged duration. It causes extensive tissue destruction and serious functional problems. E.g.: Atherosclerosis.

123. What are the causes of chronic inflammation?

- Infection E.g.: Fungi, parasites and viruses
- Prolonged exposure to toxic agents.
- Autoimmune diseases such as rheumatoid arthritis.

124. List down the morphologic features of chronic inflammation.

- Mononuclear cell infiltration, i.e, Lymphocytes, plasma cells and macrophages
- Tissue destruction
- Healing by fibrosis and angiogenesis

125. What are the factors affecting wound healing?

- Site of wound: Skin wounds heal better than wound occurring in internal organs
- Mechanical factors: Wounds at joint heal slowly if the area is not kept immobile.
- Small wound heals faster than larger wounds.

126. Define cryptorchidism.

It is the failure of testicular descends into the scrotum.

127. Define epispadiasis.

It is an abnormal opening of the urethra along the dorsal aspect of penis.

128. Define hypospadiasis.

It is an abnormal opening of the urethra along the ventral aspect of penile shaft.

129. Define fertility and infertility.

Fertilty is the ability of the person to produce offspring.

Infertility is the inability to have children.

130. Mention some venereal diseases.

- Gonorrhea
- Syphilis
- Genital Herpes

131. What is benign prostatic hyperplasia?

BPH is an enlargement of the periurethral portion of the prostate.

132. State the meaning of fibroid uterus.

It is a benign tumor arising from the smooth muscles in myometrium.

133. Define hemiplegia.

It is the condition where there is paralysis of one half of patient's body.

134. What is paraplegia?

It is an impairment in motor and loss of sensory function of the lower extremities.

135. What is meningitis?

It is an inflammation of the meninges which may be due to infection or injury.

136. What are the indications to measure prothrombin time?

- Warfarin treatment
- Liver damage
- Vitamin K status

137. Explain the abnormalities in sperm morphology.

Abnormalities may be seen in head, middle piece or tail. Macrocephaly is a presence of too large head and microcephaly is too small head. Other abnormalities are presence of double head or pointed head. The middle piece may be absent or swollen. Tail may be double, triple, rudimentary or absent.

138. How is the specimen collected for pleural or peritoneal fluid?

The sample is collected under aseptic precautions by percutaneous puncture. It is collected in 3 sterile test tubes, one containing 15mg fluoride oxalate, second containing EDTA and last is a plain tube. Examination is performed as early as possible to avoid degeneration of cells and growth of bacteria.

139. What is dipstick method?

The principle is based on the protein error of PH indicators. Tetra bromophenol blue is yellow at PH 3.0. Then it changes to bluish green in the presence of protein at the same line.

140. What is orthostatic proteinuria and Bencejone's proteinuria?

- Orthostatic proteinuria is a presence of protein in urine only when the patient is ambulatory. Hence early morning sample is negative for protein.
- Bencejone's proteinuria is seen as pathognomonic of multiple myeloma. The protein is seen in urine precipitates between 50-60 degree centigrade and sediments on boiling at 120 degree centigrade and again precipitates at 60 degree centigrade.

141. Define ulcer.

It is defined as a defect involving the epithelium. The defect may extent into the deeper connective tissue. Ulceration results from tissue necrosis and inflammation.

E.g.: Peptic ulcer of the stomach or duodenum.

142. Define inflammation.

It is a response of vascularised live tissues to injury. The injury may be caused by physical causes, chemical agents, microbes and exogenous or endogenous stimuli that disturb the normal steady state of the body.

143. Mention cells involved in inflammation.

The predominant cell of inflammation is neutrophil. Other cells are eosinophil, basophil, macrophage, platelet, lymphocytes and plasma cells.

144. What is phagocytosis?

The term phagocytosis is derived from the Greek word 'phagein' which means to eat. It is the active uptake of bacteria and cellular debris by leukocytes.

145. What are steps involved in phagocytosis?

- Recognition and attachment
- Engulfment
- Killing and degradation

146. Define malena?

Black tarry stool is seen in bleeding from the upper GI tract. This is called as malena.

147. Write the normal range of bleeding and clotting time?

- Normal bleeding time is 1-9 min.
- Normal clotting time is 5-15 min.

148. What is osteoma?

The benign bone tumors arising from the bone forming cells is called as osteoma.

149. What is rheumatoid arthritis.

RA is a chronic and systemic disease characterized by symptomatic inflammation of the joints with variable extra articular manifestations.

150. Define gout.

It is the disease characterized by elevated blood uric acid level with deposition of uric acid crystals in various tissues of the body.

151. Define quadriplegia.

It is also known as tetraplegia. It is a symptom in which a human experience paralysis affecting all the 4 limbs.

152. What are the types of stroke?

- Ischemic stroke is due to interruption of the blood supply
- Hemorrhagic stroke is due to rupture of the blood vessels

153. What is end stage glomerulopathy?

Immune mediated glomerulopathies can progress to end stage renal disease. This is also called as chronic glomerulonephritis.

154. What are the conditions where abnormal long clotting time is seen?

- Hemophilic
- Obstructive jaundice disease

155. What are the abnormal findings seen during biochemical examination of CSF?

- Protein estimation: Normal CSF protein content is 15-45 mg/dl. It is increased in all types of meningitis, subarachnoid hemorrhage and intracerebral hemorrhage
- Glucose estimation: Normal CSF glucose is 50-80 mg/dl. CSF glucose level <40mg/dl or CSF/ plasma glucose ratio < 0.3 are considered as abnormal. CSF glucose is decreased in all types of meningitis.

156. What are the findings in physical examination of pleural fluid?

Normal pleural fluid is pale straw coloured. Increased turbidity is seen in high cell count and bacterial infection. Blood tinged in pulmonary infarction and malignancy. Milky fluid is seen in tuberculosis.

157. What are contents seen in acidic urine?

Acidic urine contains?

- Uric acid and urate crystals
- Calcium oxalate
- Cystine crystals
- Tyrosine crystals
- Leucine crystals
- Sulpha crystals

158. What are contents seen in alkaline urine?

- Ammonium magnesium phosphate
- Dicalcium phosphate
- Ammonium biurate
- Calcium carbonate

159. Define tumor.

Willis defined tumor as 'an abnormal mass of tissue, the growth of which exceeds and is unco-ordinated with that of the normal tissues and persist in the same excessive manner after cessation of the stimuli.

160. Define transudate.

Inflammation is a common process that induces vascular and cellular changes. In vascular changes, the initial response of the arterioles to the injurious stimulus is vasoconstriction which last for few seconds and followed by vasodilation. Vasodilation results in an increase in blood flow causing redness, mild swelling and increase in temperature. This increased hydrostatic pressure in capillaries and venules forces a fluid through the vessel wall into the tissue. This fluid is called as transudate.

161. What are triggers of acute inflammation?

- Infections (bacterial, viral, parasitic)
- Microbial toxins
- Trauma
- Physical and chemical agents
- Foreign bodies
- Immune reactions
- Tissue necrosis

162. What are the signs of inflammation?

Cornelius Celsus (first century A.D) was the Roman physician described the 4 cardinal signs of inflammation.

- Rubor - Redness
- Calor - Heat
- Dolor - Pain
- Tumor - Swelling

163. Write two comparisons between necrosis and apoptosis.

	Necrosis	Apoptosis
1.	Cause: exogenous injury	Exogenous or endogenous injury.
2.	Mechanism; enzymatic digestion	Energy dependent genetically controlled

164. What is pyelonephritis and cystitis?

The bacterial infection of the kidney is called pyelonephritis. Infection of the urinary bladder is called cystitis.

165. Classify the calculi seen in urinary tract.

- Calcium stones
- Struvite stones or staghorn calculi
- Uric acid stones
- Cystine stones

166. What is Wilms tumor?

This is the most common solid tumor affecting infants and young children. This is also called as nephroblastoma.

167. Define azotemia.

It is elevated blood urea nitrogen and creatinine levels. This occurs due to decreased glomerular filtration rate.

168. Describe about the pathology of male genital tract.

The major problems are:

- Congenital abnormalities
- Infertility
- Inflammatory lesions
- Tumors

169. Classify testicular tumor.

1. Germ cell tumor:

- Seminoma
- Non-seminoma
- Embryonal carcinoma
- Terato carcinoma
- Chorio carcinoma
- Mixed tumor
- Teratoma
- Yolk sac tumor

2. Sex cord cell tumor

3. Metastatic tumor

170. Write the common neoplasms in female genital tract.

- Carcinoma of the cervix
- Fibroid uterus
- Carcinoma endometrium
- Ovarian tumor.

171. Write about the risk factors of cervical cancer.

- Early age at first sexual intercourse
- Multiple sexual partners
- Infection with human papilloma virus
- STD
- Cigarette smoking
- HIV infection

172. What is hydatidiform mole?

It is characterized by proliferation of the trophoblastic cells of the placenta along with hydropic degeneration of chorionic villi.

173. Write diagnostic measures of breast cancer.

- Mammography
- Fine needle aspiration cytology
- Surgical biopsy
- Lumpectomy or mastectomy.

174. What are the conditions where abnormal bleeding time occurs?

- Small blood vessel defect
- Thrombocytopenia
- Defect of platelet aggregation.

175. Describe sample collection for semen analysis.

The person should abstain from sex for a period of 3 weeks. After bladder evacuation, the sample is collected by masturbation. It is collected in a clean white mouthed screw capped container. The sample should not be stored in refrigerator. Examination should be done within 1 hour of collection.

176. Write about the physical examination of peritoneal fluid.

Normal ascetic fluid is clear and colorless. Green colour ascetic fluid is seen in poly-cystitis and gall bladder perforation. Milky ascetic fluid is seen in parasitic infection and nephritic syndrome. Hemorrhagic ascitic fluid is seen in pancreatitis, ruptured spleen and liver.

177. Explain saline preparation of stool.

A tiny sample of stool is mixed with normal saline on a glass slide and covered with a cover slip. The thickness of the sample should permit to see fine print through it. The slide is then examined under the microscope.

178. Explain iodine preparation done in stool sample for microscopy.

In this method Gram's iodine is used instead of saline. Iodine helps to visualize the nuclear structure of cysts. It stains the chromatin granules brown. The motility of parasites is not observed as iodine kills the parasite.

179. Mention two types of cell death and explain.

The two types of cell death are:

- Necrosis
- Apoptosis (Greek word- "falling off" or programmed cell death)

Necrosis is a pathologic cell death that occurs after abnormal stress and chemical injury.

Apoptosis is a form of cell death that occurs through all internally controlled suicide programme.

180. List down the differences between dry gangrene and moist gangrene.

Dry gangrene	Moist gangrene
Area affected- Limbs	Limbs and bowel
Appearance- Shriveled, gets drier and drier (mummified)	Swollen and moist
Progression- Slow	Rapid
Prognosis- Fair	Poor

181. Write down the phases of metastasis.

- Invasion of the extracellular matrix. Vascular dissemination and homing of tumor cells.

182. What are the causes of cell injury?

- Hypoxia and anoxia
- Physical agents
- Chemical agents
- Microbial pathogens
- Inflammatory mediators and immune reactions
- Genetic and metabolic disturbances
- Nutritional imbalances

183. What are the mechanisms by which substances get accumulated in the intra-cellular matrix?

- Increased production of a normal endogenous substance in the cells.
- Defective metabolism or secretion of a normal endogenous substance.

- Abnormal accumulation of an exogenous substance

184. What are the classifications of tumors?

According to the behaviour of growth, the tumours are classified into two types:

- Benign
- Malignant

Tumours are designated by attaching the suffix "oma" to the histologic cell type from which the tumour arises.

Malignant tumours of the epithelial origin are called 'carcinomas' and those of mesenchymal origin are called 'sarcomas.'

Benign tumour arising from squamous epithelium is called 'squamous papilloma.'

185. Write two comparisons of Benign and Malignant tumour.

Benign tumour	Malignant tumour
Growth- Slow, expansive, errotic with a tendency to cease.	Growth- Rapid, invasive and progressive till death
Metastasis- Never	Metastasis- Frequent
Size- Usually small	Size- Usually large
Histology- Well differentiated, well formed stroma with little tendency to haemorrhage and necrosis.	Histology- Less differentiated, anaplastic, poorly formed stroma with frequent hemorrhage and necrosis.

186. What are the risk factors of atherosclerosis?

- Modifiable risk factors - Diet, diabetes mellitus hypertension, obesity, cigarette smoking, constant stress.
- Non modifiable risk factors - Age, gender, genetic abnormalities
- Protective factors - Exercise, estrogen

187. Describe about Jones criteria.

- Pericarditis
- Polyarthritis
- Subcutaneous nodules
- Erytheme marginatum
- Chorea

188. Write the pathological causes of salmonella species.

It is caused by localized mucosal disease primarily in the ileum and the colon.

I week — Bacteremia invades

II week — Spleenomegaly and foci of necrosis in the liver

III week — Ulceration of the payers patches with intestinal bleeding and ulceration.

189. Write about the diagnosis of viral hepatitis.

Virus	Diagnosis
Hep A	Detection of serum IgM Antibodies.
Hep B	Detection of HBsAg or antibody to HBcAG
Hep C	PCR for HCV RNA-Hep D Detection of serum IgM and IgG antibodies
-Hep E	PCR for HEV RNA, Detection of serum IgM and IgG antibodies.

190. Define crescentic glomerulonephritis.

This term is used to describe severe glomerular injury accompanied by formation of xudates in the glomerular urinary space. The inflammatory cells surround the compressed capillary loops in the form of a crescent moon.

191. List down the causes of renal failure.

Pre renal causes - Hypovolemia, dehydration, poor intake of fluids, medication, eg., Lasix, obstruction of the renal artery or vein.

Renal causes - Sepsis, drugs, rhabdomyolysis (muscle breakdown), multiple myeloma

Post renal causes - Obstruction of the bladder or ureters, prostate cancer.

192. Classify testicular tumours.

- Germ cell tumours: Seminoma, Non-seminomaous, germ cell tumor, embryonal carcinoma, teratocarcinoma, choriocarcinoma, mixed tumor, teratoma, yolk sac tumor.
- Sex cord cell tumors
- Metastatic tumors

193. What is hydrocephalus?

Hydrocephalus is a term derived from the Greek words "hydro" meaning water and "cephalus" meaning head and this condition is called as "water in the brain".

194. What are tumours of the biliary hepatic system?

1. Benign tumours

-Cavernous haemangioma

-Adenoma

-Neurofibroma

-Lipoma

2. Malignant tumours

a. Primary- Hepatoma

Cholangiocarcinoma

b. Secondary sarcoma

195. What blood tests arerequired in clinical pathology?

Blood routine, hemoglobin, TC, DC, platelets, peripheral smear and MP- EDTA sample

Prothrombin time and activated partial thromboplastin time- Citrate sample

LE cell- clotted blood

Sickle cell test-EDTA blood

Osmotic fragility- Heparin

Bone marrow- EDTA blood

Factor VIII assay- Citrate sample

G6PD- EDTA sample

196. What are the findings during routine examination of semen?

Physical examination

Normal semen is gray white and viscid yellow coloured semen is seen in pyospermia. Normal volume of semen is 2-5 ml, less volume than 1.5ml is called hypospermia. Semen takes an hour to liquefy normally. Failure to liquefy indicates inadequate prostatic secretions.

Chemical examination- Normal pH of semen is 7.2- 7.8. An altered pH is seen in acute infection of prostrate, seminal vesicle and epididymis.

197. How is sample collection done for gastric and duodenal content examination?

The common method of collection is by direct brushings of visible lesions by a fibroscope. A brush enclosed in a transparent teflon sheath is passed through an endoscope. When a lesion is visualized, the brush is expelled from the sheath firmly and briskly plunged into the mucosa 5-10 times.

198. Describe the microscopy observations during stool culture.

Saline wet mount is done to demonstrate the presence of pus cells and RBCs, presence of motile trophozoites.

Iodine wet mount is done to demonstrate the presence of cysts of parasites.

GENETICS

INTRODUCTION

Transmission of characteristics from parents to children is known as heredity. The basic unit of heredity is gene, which consist of portion of DNA molecules. Genetics is the study of genes. Diagnosis of genetic condition has an impact not only the affected individuals but also their family, friends, community and society.

Cell division

Genetic information is passed from parents to all the descendent through cell division. There are two types of cell divisions, namely: mitosis, meiosis.

Chromosomes

Chromosomes appear as closed bodies and carry the hereditary materials namely genes. The normal human somatic cells contains 46 chromosomes.one set is inherited from father and the other is from mother.

Mendelian inheritance is a set of primary statements about the way certain characteristics are transmitted from parents to their offspring.

There are four patterns of inheritance:

Autosomal dominant

Autosomal recessive

X-linked dominant

X-linked recessive

Congenital anomaly

All types or anomalies or defects present at birth are termed as congenial. Birth defects can be single system defects or multiple organ syndromes.

Genetic testing

Many genetic diseases can be diagnosed by a careful history and examination of patient who is suspected to have a defect. Genetic testing is a tests to detect or exclude an alteration likely to be associated with a genetic disorder.

Genetic testing before a pregnancy is ideal, however many of the tests are done after the women becomes pregnant.

Genetherapy

Gene therapy is defined as the replacement of a deficient gene product or repair of an abnormal gene within an individual cells and tissues to treat diseases.

Genetic counselling

Genetic counselling is the process of providing clear information about the medical and family implications of a specific disease in a non-directive manner.

References

1. Nayak R, Rai S, Gupta A (2013). **Textbook of Pathology and Genetics for Nurses**. 1st ed. Jaypee
2. Kapur. (1991). **Basic Human Genetics**. 2nd ed. Jaypee.
3. Sharma S H (2001). Human Genetics in Nursing. 1st ed. Jaypee.
4. Rizwan M (2009). **Genetics Nursing Perspectives**. 1st ed. Frontline.

Test Series

1. **Mention the stages of mitosis.**
Namely it is divided into four phases
   - Prophase
   - Metaphase
   - Anaphase
   - Telophase
2. **Define fertilization.**
It is the process of union of male or female germ cells resulting in the formation of zygote. It usually occurs in the ampullary portion to the uterine tube
3. **Difference between mitosis and meiosis**
Mitosis.
   - Mitosis produces two identical cells
   - Cells created by mitosis have exactly the same number of chromosomes as the original cell did

   Meiosis:
   - Meiosis is a cell division that includes reducing the chromosome number as preparation for sexual reproduction
   - Meiosis reduces the amount of and by half so that when fertilization occurs, each offspring gets a full set of chromosomes. As a result of meiosis, the cell goes from being diploid to being haploid.
4. **What are the types of chromosomes?**
Two types of chromosomes
Sex chromosomes - These chromosomes determine gender
Autosomal chromosomes - Autosomal simply refers to non sex chromosomes
5. **How the chromosomes structures altered?**
They can be of different forms
   - Deletions
   - Duplications
   - Translocations
   - Inversions
   - Rings
   - Isochromosome
   - Chromosome instability syndrome
6. **Define mutation and its causes.**
Mutations are changes to the base pair sequence of the genetic material of an organism
Etiology:
Exposure to the ultraviolet or ionizing radiation, chemical mutations or viruses
7. **Mention the types of mutation based on the inheritance.**
   - Heterozygous mutation
   - Homozygous mutation
   - Compounds heterozygous mutation
8. **What is conditional mutation?**
Conditional mutation is a mutation that has less severe phenotype under certain permissive environmental conditions and a

mutant phenotype under certain restrictive condition

9. Differentiate maternal effect, paternal effect.

Maternal effect, in genetics, is the phenomenon where the genotype of a mother is expressed in the phenotype of its offspring unaltered by paternal genetic influence. The phenotype of an individual therefore reflects the genotype of its mother.

Paternal effect is when a phenotype results from the genotype of the father, rather than the genotype of the individual.

10. What is dominant inheritance?

A person can inherit a genetic disease when one parent (who may or may not have the disease) passes along a single faulty gene. This is called dominant inheritance. E.g.:- Achondroplasia,
Marfan syndrome.

11 What is recessive inheritance?

Genetic disease is inherited when both parents (who do not have the disease) carry an abnormality in the same gene and pass it on to a child. This is called "recessive inheritance".

E.g.:- tay-sachs disease, cystic fibrosis.

12. Give examples of multi-factorial birth defects.

- Cleft lip/palate (Opening in the lip or/ and roof of the mouth)
- Neural tube defects (Serious birth defects of the brain and spinal cord, including spina
- Bifida and anencephaly)
- Heart defects

13. What is multi-factorial inheritance?

Some birth defects appear to be caused by combination of one or more genes and environmental exposures. This is called "multi- factorial inheritance.

14. State example for metabolic disorders.

- Tay-sache disease affected babies lack an enzyme needed to break down certain fatty substances in brain cells, which results in blindness, paralysis and death.
- Phenylketonuria

15. What is FISH?

Fluoresence in situ hybridization (fish) is one technique that can be applied to aneuploid conditions such as trisomy and monosomy.

16. What does this triple screening includes?

The classic test is the triple screen for alpha fetoprotein (MS-AFP), B-HCG and Estriol [UE3]

17. What is familial cancer syndrome?

Familial cancer syndrome is a genetic condition that causes an increased risk for specific type of cancers. Familial cancer syndromes account for only 5-10 % of all cancers.

18. List the types of hemophilia.

Hemophilia types A and B.

Type A is caused by a defect in factor vii; a cofactor in the intrinsic pathway that is required for activation of the common pathway.

Type B is caused by a defect in factor ix. Type B hemophilia is sometimes called christmas disease.

19. Mention the uses for genetic testing.

Prenatal testing includes all three types of genetic testing (DNA- based, chromosome and biochemical) and is widely used for prenatal screening and diagnosis of such conditions as Down syndrome.

20. List the types of gene therapy.

- Germ line gene therapy

- Somatic cell gene therapy

21. Define genetics.

Genetics is the science of hereditary & variation in living organism

22. What is genetic code?

It is the set of rules by which information encoded in genetic material is translated into proteins by living cells

23. List the branches of genetics.

Cytogenetics, molecular genetics, developmental genetics, immunogenetics, behavioral genetics, population genetics, biochemical genetics

24. What is codon or triplet code?

The sequence of 3 bases that codes for one amino acid

25. What is the chemical composition of DNA?

- Sugar molecule
- Phosphoric acid
- Nitrogenous base
- Adenine (a), Thymine(t), Cytosine (c), Guanine (g)

26. List the 3 types of RNA.

- Messenger RNA (m RNA)
- Ribosomal RNA (r RNA)
- Transfer RNA (t RNA)

27. What is transcription?

In this process the genetic information stored in DNA (in the form of triplet code) of a gene is transmitted to messenger RNA

28. Mention the ways to prevent birth defects.

- Preconception visit with her health care provider
- Life style modifications like quitting smoking and avoiding alcohol and occupational exposures
- All pregnant ladies should take a daily multi vitamin containing 400 micro-organisms of the B-vitamin folic acid
- She should not take any medication without doctor's prescription
- She should avoid excessive contact with pets and eating low or undercooked meat

29. What is consanguinity?

Consanguinity refers to the property of being from the same lineage as another person

30. Define Atopy.

It is defined as the clinical allergies involving allergen-specific immunoglobulin . Genetic tendency to develop the classic allergic diseases such as atopic dermatitis, allergic rhinitis (hay fever) and asthma.

31. State the reasons why breast feeding reduces the occurrence of atopic diseases.

- Reduced exposure to food proteins that would be present in formulas
- Improved maturation of the intestinal barrier thereby reducing the absorption of macromolecules; reduced frequency of infection which can act as an adjuvant
- Finally, the presence of anti-inflammatory factors and anti-idiotypic in human breast milk

32. List the tests used to detect major birth defects.

- Triple marker screening
- Ultrasound
- Amniocentesis

33. Mention the teratogenic agents.

Ionizing radiation, infections, metabolic imbalances, drugs and environmental chemicals

34. List the classification of genetic disease.

- Single gene disease
- Multifactorial disease
- Chromosomal disorders
- Somatic genetic disorder

35. Mention some genetic tests.
Fluorescence in situ hybridization (fish), High resolution metaphase banding technique.

36. List the types of haemochromatosis.
- Haemochromatosis types 1-3 are inherited in an autosomal recessive fashion.
- Haemochromatosis type 4 is inherited in an autosomal dominant fashion.

37. What is the gilles de la taurette syndrome?
This is a rare syndrome characterized by motor and vocal ties and sometimes involving coprolalia (use of foul language).
It may be due to an autosomal dominant gene.

38. Mention the types of genetic test used for the diagnosis of down syndrome Huntington disease; hereditary breast/ovarian cancer, sickle cell anemia.
- **Down syndrome**: Chromosomal analysis.
- **Huntington disease:** DNA analysis
- **Hereditary breast/ovarian cancer:** DNA analysis.
- **Sickle- cell anemia**: Hemoglobin electrophoresis

39. What is gene therapy?
Gene therapy is the insertion of genes into an individual's cells and tissues to treat a disease and hereditary disease in which a defective instant allele is replaced with functional gene.

40. What is isochromosomes?
A new type of chromosome may arise from a medical division at the centromere,the centromere divides perpendicular to the long axis of the chromosome understood of parallel to it.

41. List the major divisions in genetics.
- Classical Genetics
- Molecular Genetics
- Population Genetics
- Quantitative Genetics

42. List some chromosomal aberrations affecting autosomes.
- Down syndrome
- Edward's syndrome
- Patau's syndrome.

43. What is frame shift mutation?
The deletion or insertion of a base leads to an alteration in the reading frame of DNA strand and thus the amino acid sequence.

44. What is "base pair rule"?
- Adenine pairs with thymine
- Guanine pairs with cytosine.

45. Define alleles.
Alternative forms of gene at the same locus on homologous chromosomes

46. Define karyotyping.
It is the process by which the metaphase chromosomes obtained for analysis and photographed. Photographs of individual chromosomes are cut and arranged according to standard classification

47. What is non-obstructive azoospermia (NOA)?
NOA is defined as zero sperm count in the ejaculate due to sperm production problem within the testicular tissue

48. What is zoospermia?
Obstructive azoospermia is defined as zero sperm count in the ejaculate secondary to a blockage within the reproductive tract.

49. What is klinefelter syndrome?
It means the patients are phenol typically males but show presence of sex chromatin (47 XXY).

50. What is a gene mutation?
Gene mutation is a change in an organism's genetic material. Gene mutations can occur

for a variety of reasons, and have a range of effects, from benign to malignant.

51. List down the types of mutation.

- substitution
- Insertion
- Deletion
- Frame shift

52. Define turner syndrome.

Turner syndrome is a genetic condition in which a female does not have the usual pair of two X chromosomes.

53. Mention the tests performed to diagnose turner syndrome.

- Blood hormone levels (luteinizing hormone and follicle stimulating hormone)
- Echocardiogram
- Karyotyping
- MRI of the chest
- Ultrasound of reproductive organs and kidneys
- Pelvic exam
- Turner syndrome may also alter various estrogen levels in the blood and urine.

54. Define marfan syndrome.

Marfan syndrome is a disorder of connective tissue, the tissue that strengthens the body's structures. Disorders of connective tissue affect the skeletal system, cardiovascular system, eyes, and skin.

55. What causes marfan's syndrome?

Marfan syndrome is caused by a defect in the gene that encodes the structure of fibrillin and the elastic fibers, a major component of connective tissue. This gene is called fibrillin-1 or FBN1

56. What is mutation testing?

Mutation testing involves deliberately altering a program's code, then re-running a suite of valid unit tests against the mutated program. A good unit test will detect the change in the program and fail accordingly.

57. What is Down syndrome?

Down syndrome is a genetic condition in which a person has 47 chromosomes instead of the usual 46.

58. Mention the characteristics of a baby with down syndrome.

Head and facial features:

- Flattened back of head.
- Attractive Almond-shaped eyes, with one eye lid a little droopy.
- Slightly flattened bridge across nose.
- Smallish ears, positioned slightly lower on the head, with a small fold at the top of the ear.
- Smallish mouth.
- Slightly protruding tongue.

Hand feature:

- Horizontal crease in palm of hand.
- Slightly shortened fingers.
- The little finger curves inward.

Foot features :

- Slightly enlarged gap between the big and second toes.
- Slightly shortened toes.

59. What is mutation?

Any change in sequence of genomic DNA is called as mutation

60. State Mendel's laws.

- Law of inheritance
- Law of segregation
- Law of independent assortment

61. What is polyploidy?

Multiples of haploid set of chromosomes

62. Name two autosomal dominant inheritance.

Rh blood group, congenital cataract, myotonic dystrophy

63. Name 2 autosomal recessive inheritance.

Microcephaly, albinism, sickle cell anemia, schizophrenia

64. Describe the achievements of fertilization.

Reconstitution of species specific chromosomes

Allows for biparental inheritance Initiation of cleavage

65. Explain telocentric chromosomes.

They have a centromere at one end and have only one arm. It is associated with small round structures called satellites.

66. State the mechanism of inactivation of X chromosome.

X-inactivation (lyonization) is a process by which one of the two copies of the X chromosome present in female is inactivated. The inactive X chromosome is silenced by packaging into transcriptionally inactive heterochromatin. X-inactivation occurs so that the female, with two X chromosomes, does not have twice as many X chromosome gene products as the male, which only possess a single copy of the X chromosome

67. Mention 2 types of spina bifida.

- Spina bifida occulta
- Spina bifida cystica

68. Mention some genetic tests.

- Fluorescence in situ hybridization (fish)
- High resolution metaphase bonding technique

69. Mention some teratogens.

- Ionizing radiation
- Chemical teratogens

70. List some prenatal diagnostic test.

- Ultrasonography
- Aminocentesis
- Maternal blood sampling

71. Mention the major reason for the spontaneous abortions.

Chromosomal abnormalities and major birth defects

72. What is turner's syndrome?

The female patients with ovarian dysgenesis have 45 chromosome with only a single X and chromatin negative

73. Mention some clinical features of Huntington's disease.

- Chorea
- Dementia
- Hypotonicity

74. What is genetic haemochromatosis?

Autosomal dominant disorder leads to excessive iron absorption

75. Define familial cancer.

Familial cancer syndrome is genetic condition that causes an increased risk for specific type of cancer

76. List the predisposing syndrome of familial cancer.

- Adenomatous polyposis
- Retinoblastoma
- Multiple endocrine neoplasia

77. List ethics of genetic counselling.

- Providing adequate knowledge about the condition
- Counsellor should not force his ideas on patient

78. What is euthenics?

Improving human race by improving the environment

79. What happens in sister chromatid exchange?

It involves crossing over between the sister chromatids of a single chromosomes in mitosis. It was first demonstrated in 1957 by Taylor. In this technique the cultured cells are allowed to replicate twice in the presence of bromodeoxyuridine.

80. What occurs in second meiotic division of oogenesis?

The female germ cell passes into the uterine tube, but is not completed until after fertilization.

81. What is g-banding?

Slides with chromosomes preparation are first treated with a solution of trypsin, and after denatures the chromosome protein and stained with giemsa solution. It shows dark and light bands

82. What is splice mutation?

These affect a normal mechanism by which introns are excised and exons are spliced together during the formation of a messenger RNA. It leads complete failure of the gene product.

83. What is the meaning of the symbol DEL, DUP and INV?

Deletion, duplication, inversion

84. Which type of test is required for repeated foetal loss?

Karyotype analysis of both partners

85. What is the applications of DNA finger printing technology?

- Used in forensic science
- Number of genetic disorders can be recognized before the onset
- Tissue matching can be done
- Gene locations can be found

86. What is northern blotting?

Northern blotting involves the use of electrophoresis to separate RNA samples by capillary transfer of RNA from the electrophoresis gel to the blotting membrane called as first blotting technique

87. What is lyon hypothesis?

In the normal female one of the two X chromosomes is randomly inactivated and appears in somatic cells as sex chromatin

88. What is meant by simian crease?

A single palmer occurs in down syndrome is called simian crease

89. List the types of translocation.

- Robertsonian translocation
- Reciprocal translocation

90. What is ring chromosome?

It involves two breaks at the terminal portions of the chromosome followed by fusion of cut ends.

91. What is the cytogenetics of down syndrome?

Individuals show translocation (14q21q). Long arm of chromosome 21 is translocated to long arm of chromosome 14.

92. What is true hermaphrodite?

A true hermaphrodite has ambiguous genitalia of varying degree. It ranges from individuals who appear to be almost like a normal male to those who appear almost like a female.

93. Mention three gene families so far identified in vertebrates.

Homeobox (hox) genes, paired box genes and zinc finger genes.

94. What is pleiotropy?

When a single gene or a gene pair produces multiple phenotypic effects, it is called pleiotropy.

95. What is Gower's sign?

When child wants to rise from the floor, the child attempts it by pushing on or climbing up his legs and thighs, it is called gower's sign.

96. What is the management of duchene muscular dystrophy?

- Direct injection of recombinant DNA

- Myoblast implantation
- Transfection with retroviral or adeno-viral vectors containing a dystrophin minigene

97. State the problems and ethics of gene therapy.
- Short lived nature of gene therapy
- Immune response
- Problem with viral vectors
- Multi gene disorders
- Chance of inducing a tumor
- Religious concerns
- Death

98. Mention the goals of human genome project.

To identify approximate 20,000-25,000 genes sequence of 3 billion chemical base pairs etc

PHARMACOLOGY

INTRODUCTION

Pharmacology is the study of drugs. Drugs are chemicals that produce therapeutically useful effects. Drugs are an essential part of treatment of illness. Safe use of drugs requires sound knowledge of:

Mode of action

Side effects

Dosage

Rate and route of administration

Interactions

Drugs are obtained from plants, animals, microbes and mineral sources.

Pharmacodynamics

Pharmacodynamics is the study of drug effects and their mechanisms of action. It mainly includes;

Study of biological and therapeutic effects

The mechanisms of action

Correlation of drug action with chemical structure

Pharmacokinetics

Pharmacokinetics is the quantitative study of drug movement through and out of the body. It is a study of absorption, distribution, metabolism and excretion of drugs.

Routes and principles of drug administration

The drugs may be administered locally or administered systemically based on the nature of the drug and the patient. Common routes of administration of drugs are: Topical, oral, transdermal, rectal, inhalation and parenteral.

Rights of drug administration

The traditional five rights of drug administration are: Right patient, right drug, right dose, right route and right time.

Chemotherapy

Chemotherapy is the use of chemicals in infectious diseases to destroy microorganisms, without damaging the host tissues. Antibiotics are substances produced by microorganisms which suppress the growth of or destroy other pathogens.

Antiseptics, disinfectants and insecticides

In hospitals, standard cleaning procedures reduces the number of pathogens by removing the threat of infection. Hence disinfection is the suitable procedure. There are agents which inhibit or kill microorganisms on contact. 1. Antiseptics, 2. Disinfectants

These drugs act by oxidation of bacterial protoplasm and denaturation of bacterial proteins which is a detergent like action increasing permeability of bacterial membrane.

References

1. Sudhakar, GK,. (2010). **Pharmacology for Nurses**. 1st ed. Jypee.
2. Tripathi KO (2003). **Essentials of Pharmacology for Nurses**. 5th ed. Jypee.
3. Padmaja U (2008). **Pharmacology for Nursing.** 2nd ed. Jypee.

Test Series

1. **What is pharmacology?**
   The word pharmacology is derived from Greek words 'pharmacon' and 'logos.' 'Pharmacon' means an 'active principles' and 'logos' means a 'discourse.'
   Pharmacology is the science that deals with drugs. It consists of detailed study of drugs particularly their action on living organisms
2. **Mention the objectives of pharmacology.**
   The object of pharmacology is mainly to provide such scientific data, using which one can choose a drug treatment of proven efficacy and safety from the various options available to suit the patient
3. **Define drug.**
   The word drug is derived from the French word 'drogue' means 'A dry herb'.
   According to WHO "A drug is any substance or product that is used or intended to be used to modify or explore physiological systems or pathological stats for the benefit of the recipient"
4. **What is clinical pharmacy?**
   Clinical pharmacy involves cooperation of the pharmacist with physician in educating the patient about complaints and counselling him on how to take medication and monitoring for errors in drug therapy
5. **What is pharmacokinetics?**
   Pharmacokinetics is the study of the absorption, distribution, metabolise and excretion of drugs and their relationship to pharmacological response
6. **What is pharmaco dyanamics?**
   The quantitative study of the biological and therapeutic effects of drugs
7. **What is therapeutics?**
   Therapeutics means 'to care for', 'to tend to', 'to nurse' and it is a branch of medicine concerned with a cure of disease or relief of symptoms.
8. **What is toxicology?**
   Toxicology is the science of poisons which includes detection and measurement of poisons as well as treatment of poisoning.
9. **Define chemotherapy.**
   Chemotherapy concerned with an effect of drugs upon micro-organisms and parasites living and multiplying in a living organisms.
10. **What is pharmaco epidemiology?**
    Pharmaco epidemiology is the study of the use and the effects of the drugs in large number of people. It helps to gain further insight into the efficacy and safety of new drugs after they are released.
11. **What is pharmaco ecomonics?**
    It is the analysis of the cost of drug therapy to the health care system and the society.

12. What is pharmaco vigilence?
The process of identifying and responding to the issues of drug, safety to the detection of drug effects usually adverse.

13. Define pharmaco genetics.
It is the study of inherited variations mediated through single gene in drug metabolism and response in humans.

14. What is pharmaco genomics?
The science that examines the heritable variation in genes that dictate the drug response of humans and microbes.

15. What is pharmacopeia?
It is an official code containing the selected list of the essential drugs and the medicinal preparations with prescriptions of physical properties and rest of their identity, purity and potency.

16. What are the natural sources of drugs?
They are mineral, animal, plant, microorganisms, synthetic, genetic engineering and hybridoma techniques

17. What are the main routes of administration of drugs?
Topical, oral, sublingual, rectal, parenteral and pulmonary (inhalation) routes.

18. What is drug bio availability?
It indicates the overall proportions of the drug that passes into the systemic circulation after its administration. It is defined as the rate and extent to which therapeutic moiety becomes available to the site of drug action.

19. What is zero order kinetics?
It is the amount changed per unit time is constant. Hence zero order elimination kinetics means the amount of drug eliminated per unit time is constant.

20. What are advantages of parenteral routes?

- Can be employed in unconscious and un cooperative patients
- Can be employed in case of vomiting and diarrhoea
- Drugs which might irritate the stomach or which are not absorbed orally can be administrated
- They avoid drug modification by the alimentary juices and liver enzyme
- Rapid action and accuracy

21. What is therapeutic index?
Dose which produces a defined unwanted effect (e.g.: tachycardia) in 50% of the test subjects. Dose producing therapeutic effect (specified reduction in air way resistance) in 50% of the test subjects

22. Specify the antidotes for cyanide poisoning.
Dicobalt edentate, amyl nitrite followed by sodium nitrate, then sodium thio-sulfate

23. Write principles of de addiction.

- Hospitalization of patient
- Gradual or sudden withdrawal of the drug
- Substitution therapy
- Psychotherapy and occupational therapy
- Specific drug therapy e.g,; Disulfiram in alcohol addiction
- Correction of nutritional deficiencies
- Community treatment and rehabilitation

24. Name the agents used in the treatment of hypocalcemia.

- Prednisolone
- Plicamycin
- Calcitonin
- Disodium edentate
- Sodium pyruvate to reduce absorption from gut.

25. What is streptokinase?
Streptokinase is a non-enzymatic protein derived from beta-hemolytic streptococci. It complexes with plasminogen to liberate

plasmin.

Uses

- For acute myocardial infarction within 3 to 4 hours of the onset of pain.
- In pulmonary embolism
- For venous thrombo-embolism
- For deep vein thrombosis (DVT)

26. What is drug tolerance?

- Natural tolerance
- Acquired tolerance
- Cross tolerance

27. What are drug receptors?

The receptor is a component of a cell with a chemical agent. It has domains, ligand binding effectors domain.

28. List the factors affecting oral drug absorption and bioavailability.

A) **Drug related**: Physical properties of the drug, nature of the dosage, forms.

B) **Patient related**: Physiological factors, pharmacogenetic factors, diseased states.

29. What is the emergency treatment of acute drug poisoning?

- Check for ABG
- Gastric lavage
- Activated charcoal
- Dialysis
- Antidote
- IV Glucose
- Follow up

30. What is effect of food on drug absorption?

Food aids the absorption of chloroquine, carbamezipine, griseofulvin, lithium carbonate, riboflavin, and spironolactone.

31. What is intrathecal administration?

Introduction of drugs such as spinal anesthetics into the subarachnoid space. The drug acts on CNS. Eg., anti malignancy drugs.

32. How are the drugs distributed in different body parts?

Total body water, extra cellular space, intravascular space, body fat, bones. Types of drugs are water soluble molecules, strongly protein bound molecules and highly liquid soluble molecules.

33. What is blood brain barrier?

The composition of the CSF and the extra cellular fluid in the brain differs significantly from that of the plasma. A specialized system that fluctuates the composition of the plasma and protects the brain from toxic substances.

34. What is esterification?

Steroidal sex hormones such as testosterones and estrogens, when esterified with carboxylic acids, gives compounds such as benzoate, propionate, ennthate which are absorbed slowly.

35. What is the ocusert?

Ocusert, when placed under the eyelid can deliver a steady flow of pilocarpine round the clock for 7 days without causing any discomfort thus avoiding the need for repeated eye drops.

36 What is the important allergic reactions to penicillin?

The reactions are skin rashes, arthritis, serum sickness like syndrome, renal disturbances, hemopoietic disturbances, angioedema and anaphylaxis

37. Write down the guiding principles for the use of cephalosporins.

- Cephalosporins are expensive and should not be used where an equally effective, alternative antibiotic is available
- None of them is effective against infections by enterococci

- None of them is agent of choice against anaerobic infection

38. Write the therapeutic uses of aminoglycosides.

- Topical use in the eye and on the skin-neomycin, framycetin, gentamicin
- GI Infections and gut sterilization: Neomycin, paromomycin
- Systemic use –sterptomycin, gentamycin, kanamycin, amikacin, netilmicin

39. Write action mechanism of macrolides.

Macrodides act by inhibiting the protein synthesis by binding to the 50S ribosomal subunits

40. Write about the absorption of sulphonamides.

Sulphonamides intended for systemic use are rapidly absorbed from the GI tract and 70-90% of the oral dose reaches the blood stream. The main site of absorption is the small intestine.

41 What is the mechanism of action of quinolones?

The activity of quinolones against gram positive bacteria is primarily due to their action of DNA gyrase. Whereas that against gram positive bacteria is primarily due to their action on topoisomerase.

42. Classify drugs for tuberculosis.

Rifampicin, isoniazid, pyrazinamide, streptomycin, ethambutol, thiocetazone.

43. What are the drugs used for viral infections?

Idoxuridina, acyclovir, ganciclovir, adefovir, lamivudine, ribovirin.

44. Write commonly used anti helminthic drugs.

- Albendazole
- Metronidazole
- Praziquante
- Metrifonate
- Piperazine

45. Write down the adverse reactions of metronidazole.

Vomiting, vertigo, headache, diarrhoea, abdominal pain, pruritis and flushing. Mild blood dyscrasis, seizures, ataxia.

46. Write WHO recommended regimen for leprosy.

Leprosy Type	Drugs	Duration
Tuberculoid	Dapsone (100mg)	6 months
	Rifampicin (600mg	
Lepromatous	Dapsone (100mg)	12 months
	Clofazimine (50mg)	
	Rifampicin (600mg)	6 months

47. Write action mechanism of chloroquine.

Malarial parasite digests Hb in their lysosomes to utilize amino acids. Chloroquine being the basic drug concentrate in their acidic lysosomes and binds to liberated heme.

48. List down immuno suppressants.

- T cell inhibitors – Cyclosporine,
- Glucocorticoid – Prednisolone,
- Cytotoxic agents – Azathioprine.

49. What are the drugs that should be avoided in pregnancy?

Anti- tubercular drugs: e.g, streptomycin (causes deafness), pyrazinamide (teratogenic drugs)

50. Write the various drug regimens in the treatment of tuberculosis.

- Short course chemotherapy.

Daily regimen – 6 to 9 months
Intermittent regimen – 9 months
2. Long term chemotherapy- 18 months.

51. Write the treatment for UTI with dosage.
- Sulfisoxazole 2g
- Amoxicillin 3g
- Ciprofloxczine 250 – 500 mg,
- Carbemicillin indanyl 2 tab

52. List the drugs effective for typhoid fever.
- Chloramphenicol
- Ciprofloxacin
- Cotrimexazone
- Ampicillin
- Third Generation Cephalosporin.

53. State the role of nurses in administration of rifampicin.
Assess allergic reactions; inform the patients that the urine, faeces, saliva, sputum, sweats may turn orange red.

54. Which antitubercular drugs should be avoided in pregnancy and why?
- Streptomycin (It causes deafness)
- Pyrazinamide (A teratogenic drug)
- Long term chemotherapy – drugs which are given for 18 months

55. Write the mechanism of action of disinfectants and antiseptics.
- Coagulation of the bacterial proteins
- An alternation in the properties of bacterial cell wall
- Binding of the free sulfhydryl
- Competition with essential subtracts for the important enzymes in the bacterial cell

56. Mention the gaseous type of disinfectant.
Methylene oxides, metapropiolacton in the gaseous form are powerful agents. It is colourless liquid with boiling point

57. Specify common insecticides. Who discovered the drug.
DDT was first highly effective And relatively safe insecticides discovered by Muller who was later awarded the Nobel prize for medicine in 1948.

58. What is surfactants?
It lowers surface tension of solution, usually aqueous forms. They are termed as detergents.

59. State examples of disinfectants.
Salicylic acid sodium and potassium hydroxide, phenol, formaldehyde.

60. Give examples of insecticides.
DDT, carbaryl, malathion, parathion.

61. What are the uses of oxidizing agent?
- Used for cleaning wounds, abscess
- For removal of adhering dressings
- Irrigations
- Used in mouth wash

62. What are the types of radiation?
- Non ionizing radiation- Infra red radiation, ultraviolet radiation.
- Ionizing radiation- Gamma rays.

63. Describe hot air oven?
It is commonly used to dry sterilized glass syringes and instruments. It is carried out at 160 degree Celsius to 180 degree Celsius for 60-120 min,

64. Name the chemical methods of high level disinfection.
Sodium hypochlorite, Chloramine T, Ethanol, Cetrimide, Povidone iodine, Formaldehyde, Glutaraldehyde, Hydrogen peroxide.

65. Classify antiemetic drugs.
- Antidopaminergic e.g. Chlorpromazine
- Antihistaminic e.g. Promethazine, cyclizine
- Antimuscarinic e.g. Scopolamine
- Anti-5 HT e.g. Ondandsetron
- Antagonistic of the NKI receptors for substance P
- Miscellaneous such as Nabilone, tri-

methobenzamide, benzquinamide

66. List drugs which cause diarrhoea.

- Magnesium antacids
- Antibiotics: erythromycin, ampicillin, tetracycline
- GI-Prokinetic drugs
- Quinidine
- Prostaglandin analogous
- Colchicine
- Emetine
- Cytotoxic drugs
- Lithium

67. Classify antacids.

- Non systemic antacids. E.g.: Aluminium hydroxide gel
- Systemic Antacids. E.g.: Sodium bicarbonate.

68. What are the main sites of action of acetyl choline?

Preganglionic fibres, autonomic ganglion, post ganglionic fibres, neuro muscular junction.

69. Write the pharmacological management of peptic ulcer.

Antacids: Aluminum hydroxide gel, sodium bicarbonate

- Anti-secretory agents Proton pump inhibitor
- H2 receptor antagonist
- Mucosal protective agents; Bismuth salts.

70. Name drugs which produce constipation.

Anti cholinergics, anti histaminic, anti parkinsonian, antipsychotics, anti- depressants.

71. State the management of constipation.

- Irritant laxatives, e.g.: Anthraquinone,
- Osmotic laxatives, e.g.: Lactulose,
- Bulk laxatives, e.g.: Methyl cellulose, agar,
- Emollient laxatives, e.g. Liquid paraffin

72. Mention contraindication of purgatives.

- Undiagnosed acute abdomen
- Intestinal obstruction
- Stimulant purgatives are avoided during pregnancy

73. List the side effects of metaclopromide.

Drowsiness, dizziness, dystonic reaction, diarrhoea, gynaecomastia, galactorrhoea, malignant neuroleptic syndrome, parkinsonism

74. Name some hepatotoxic drugs.

Halothane, rifampicin, isoniazid, chlorpromazine, erythromycin estolate, paracetamol.

75. What is sucralfate?

Sucralfate is a complex formed from sucrose, octasulfate and poly aluminium hydroxide.

76. What is an expectorant (mukinetic agent)?

"Expectorate"- in Latin word meaning 'to drive from the chest.' E.g.: ammonium chloride, ammonium citrate, potassium iodide,. glyceryl quaiacolate

77. Name few mucolytic drugs.

Bromhexine, acetylcysteine and pancreatic dornase - they make the sputum thin and less viscid. So that it can be easily expectorated

78. What is the role of methotrexate in bronchial asthma?

Low dose methotrexate is used in the management of steroid dependent asthma by stabilizing the disease and allowing reduction in corticosteroid dosage.

79. Name some anti-tussives.

Opiates like codeine, non opioids like carbetapentane, anti-histamines like hydramine, local anaesthetics like benzoate

80. How does corticosteroid help in status asthmaticus?

They act as antiinflammatory agents. They inhibit the synthesis of eicosanoids and lymphokines. They stabilize the lysosomal membrane and prevent the mediators of inflammation.

81. Mention the drugs known to cause bronchospasm.

Aspirin, and other NSAIDs, beta adrenergic blockers, cholinergic drugs, quinine, morphine.

82. What will happen if aminophylline is given rapidly by intravenous route?

Rapid IV administration of aminophylline may result in sudden death due to cardiac arrhythmias. So diluted solution is injected slowly IV over 25-30 minutes to avoid severe toxic symptoms like headache, palpitation, hypotension, tachycardia

83. Mention types of inhalers and its action.

- Pressurized metered dose aerosol inhalers
- Dry powders inhalers
- Nebulization

Action: Relaxes the smooth muscles, enhances mucociliary clearances, suppress micro vascular leakage in the air way, inhibit release of acetyl choline

84 List the sideeffects of salbutmol.

Tremors, headache, palpitation are the main side effects of salbutomol.

85. What is the current therapy of COPD?

It includes

- Inhaled glucocorticoids
- Inhaled bronchodilators
- Oxygen inhalation
- Physiotherapy
- Pulmonary rehabilitation

86. What are the drugs that should be avoided in status asthmatics? Why?

Sedatives, tranquillizers and antihistamines are avoided because the patient gets drowsy and aggravate anoxia. Morphine is also contraindicated as it constricts the bronchi and depresses the respiratory centre.

87. How does mannitol act?

Mannitol, a non electrolyte of low molecular weight, not metabolized in the body, is freely filtered at the glomerulus and undergoes limited reabsorption. As the fluid in the proximal tubule is osmotic, the osmotic pressure exerted by mannitol limits water reabsoption

Passive reabsorption of Na+ and Cl- is decreased. Manntiol also tends to increase glomerular filtration rate by expanding plasma volume

88. What are the adverse effects of thiazides?

- Hypokalemia, hyponatremia, hypochloremia, hypotension,
- Hypoglycemia
- Hypouricemia
- Hyperlipidemia
- Renal insufficiency may be aggregated in patients with decreased renal reserve
- Hypersensitivity reactions
- GI disturbances-nausea, vomiting, diarrhoea, pancreatitis
- Impotence reduced libido

89. What is meant by high ceiling diuretics?

Peak diuresis produced by high ceiling diuretic is for greater than observed with other diuretics. They have distinctive action on renal tubular function.

90. What are the therapeutic uses of spironolactone?

Refractory edema associated with secondary hyperaldosteronism. To counteract potassium loss due to thiazides, resistant hypertension, hirrsutism, hyperglycemia, hyperurecemia, hypokalemia.

91. Why diuretics should not be used in toxemia of pregnancy?

In pregnancy, blood volume is low in spite of edema. Diuretics further decrease it and compromise placental circulation and may lead to miscarriage, fetal death.

92. What is the treatment for acidosis?

Slow infusion of 7.5% sodium bicarbonate to improve the plasma bicarbonate concentration.

93. Mention the treatment for alkalosis.

IV normal saline in acute alkalosis

In chronic cases potassium loss need to be rectified. e.g.: KCl (Inj /syrup)]

94. State the indications of total parental nutrition.

Short bowel syndrome, pancreatic abscess, alimentary tract cancer, crohn's disease.

95. Mention the adverse effects of thiazides.

Hyponatremia, hypokalemia, hypochloremia, hypotension, hyperglycemia, hypophospotemia

96. List the factors affecting plasma potassium.

- Potassium intake
- Total body sodium
- Acidosis and alkalosis
- Changes in the cell metabolism
- Hormones
- Drugs are the factors affecting plasma potassium.

97. Mention the treatment for cirrhotic edema and ascites.

- Bed rest
- Restriction of sodium intake-20mEq/day
- Oral potassium supplements
- Spironolactone

98. Describe the symptoms of alcohol withdrawal.

Alcohol craving, tremor, irritability, nausea, sleep disturbances, tachycardia, hypotension, sweating, seizures 12-24 hrs after the last drink delirium tremens (confusion, visual hallucinations, fever, profuse sweating)

99. Describe the symptoms of nicotine withdrawl.

Irritability, impatience, hostility, anxiety, depressed mood, difficulty in concentrating, restlessness, increased heart rate, increased appetite

100. What are three general principles of suppression?

- Primary immune responses can be more easily & more effectively suppressed than secondary immune responses
- Immunosuppressive agents do not produce the same effects on all immune response
- Inhibition of the immune response is more likely to occur if the immunosuppressive therapy is begin before, rather than after exposure to immunogen.

101. Name some immunosuppressive agents.

- Cyclosporin
- **Cytotoxic agents** – Azathioprine, methotrexate, cyclophosphamide
- **Antibodies** – Lymphocyte immunoglobulins, mono clonal antibody to CD3
- **Other agents** – Adrenocorticosteroids, sulfasalazine, thalidomide

102. What is the mechanism of action cyclosporine?

Cyclosporine is a peptic antibiotic. It has selective ability to inhibit activation of T cells. It inhibits an early response to antigenic and regulatory stimuli primarily in T helper cells.

103. How does methotrexate act as animmuno supressants?

It inhibits replication and function of T cells and B cells, because of a selective action on DNA synthesis.

104. What are the therapeutic uses of antibodies on immuno suppressants?

Lymphocyte Ig is used in acute graft rejection and aplastic anemia, monoclonal antibodies used as adjuvants in acute rejection of the renal allograft.

105. What is passive immunization?

Here performed antibodies of human or animal origin is used to transfer immunity to host.

106. Name some specific products used for passive immunization.

Diphtheria anti toxin, snake and spider anti- venom, immunoglobulin for hepatitis B, pertussis, rabies, tetanus, varicella. Their half life is 5-7 days.

107. Name a few attenuated immunogens.

Vaccines for measles, mumps, rubella and polio.

108. Name a few common drug interactions of vitamin B 6.

INH is prevented by pyridoxine. INH inhibits enzymatic reactions in which pyridoxine is a coenzyme and increases urinary excretion of vitamin B 6.

109. What is overdosage toxicity of ascobic acid?

Oxalate renal stones.

110. Name few vitamins which protect against cancer.

Vitamin A protects against skin cancer
Vitamin C and E inhibit formation of carcinogens

111. What are toxic effects of vitamin K?

- Rapid IV injection of emulsified vitamin K may produce flushing, breathlessness, fall in BP, death
- Menadione and its water soluble derivatives can cause hemolysis in patients with G6 PD deficiency are more susceptible
- In newborns kernicterus may be precipitated due to hemolysis and competitive inhibition of glucuronidation of bilirubin

112. Name the drugs used in the treatment of hypercalcemia.

Prednisolone, plicamycin, calcitonin, disodium edetate, sodium pyruvate.

113. What is dihydro tachysterol?

It is the product of calciferol, it raises plasma calcium but has anthracitic activity. Its action is faster and shorter lived. It mobilizes calcium from bone, decreases absorption from gut and promotes urinary excretion of calcium.

114. Name some compounds useful in paget's disease of bones?

- Calcitonin
- Mithramycin
- Sodium ethidronate
- Sodium pamidronate
- Alendronate

115. What are the uses of nicotinic acid?

Pellagra - prophylaxis and treatment
Carcinoid syndrome

116. What is overdosage toxicity of ascorbic acid? What is its normal dosages with its therapeutic uses?

Toxicity leads to oxalate renal stones
Normal dosage is 50 mg, Ascorbic injection: dose-0.1-1gm IM or IV
Therapeutic uses

- Scurvy
- Methemoglobinemia

- Multivitamin combinations

117. Mention the antidotes for carbon monoxide poisoning.

Hyperbaric oxygen, dandrolene, sodium bi carbonate carbamazepine, dapsone, phenobarbital, quinine, salicylate and colchicine

118. What are emollients?

These preparations increased the water content of stratum corneum by forming an occlusive film that prevents normal transepidermal water loss. This result in softening of skin and a decrease in scaling, cracking and fissuring

119. What is keratolysis and give some example of keratolytics?

They cause of peeling of superficial layers of skin. They are used to destroy unwanted tissues like warts and callus. E.g: Trichloroacetic acid, silver nitrate, salicyclic acid, propylene glycol. Benzyl peroxide and tretinoin are used in acne

120. Name the drugs used in the treatment of psoriasis.

Anti-mitotic, topical adrenal steroids, calcipotriol, etretinate, psoralin, methotrexate, cyclosporine.

121. Name an agent which can protect against photo sensitivity.

Chloroquine, acts systemically used agent which protect against photosensitivity.

122. What are harmful effects of UV light?

UVA (320-440) causes skin cancer and skin ageing. UVB (290-320) nm causes sun burn and skin cancer for ageing. UVC (200-290) nm causes skin injury at high altitude.

123. Name the drugs which can produce photosensitivity.

Systematically used drugs such as Sulfonamides, frusemide, thiazide diuretics, sulfonylurea agents, tetracyclines, griseofulvin, phenothiazine, nalidoxic acid, oral contraceptives, chlorodiazepoxide, amiodarone, piroxicam

Topically applied substance: Deodorants, hexachlorophene, para-aminobenzoic acid, coal-tar derivatives

124. How are warts treated?

Cryotherapy, salicylic acid, 12%, salicylic acid and lactic acid paint or gel.Formaldehyde or glutaraldehyde, podophyllin for plantar anogenital warts

125. State the guidelines for topical corticosteroids.

- Use weakest preparation to control the disorder
- In resistant cases, use a high potency preparation for a short (3 wks) period
- Apply thin film
- Give small quantity
- Occlusive dressing used for a brief period.

126. Mention the drug therapy for herpes simplex and herpes zoster.

5% Acyclovir or 1% penciclovir

Idoxuridine, carbamazepine, gabapentine.

127. Name the drugs that should be discontinued prior to surgery.

Combined oral contraceptive pill (4 weeks), MAOIs (2 weeks), lithium (2 days) and aspirin (1 week) before surgery to be stopped. On the other hand, drugs like glucocorticoids, analgesics, anti parkinsonian drugs, antiglucoma drugs, thyroid and antithyroid drugs should be continued

128. What are the three cardinal features of general anaesthesia?

- Unconsciousness
- Analgesia
- Loss of motor reflexes

129. What is mechanism and site if action of

benzodiazepine?

Mechanism of action:

Benzodiazepines bind to benzodiazepine/ GABA receptor which leads to increase in chloride conductance.

Site: receptors are located in cerebral cortex, mid brain, reticular formation, limbic system, cerebellum and spinal cord. They potentiate the neural inhibition mediated by GABA at all levels of neurotoxin

130. Name the classical (typical) antipsychotic drugs.

- Phenothiazines
- Aliphatic - Chlorpromazine, promazine
- Piperazine - Fluphenazine, trifluroperazine
- Piperazine - hioridazine
- Butyrophenones - Haloperidol, droperidol, benperidol, trifluperidol
- Thioxanthenes - Flupenthixol, clopenthixol

131. What is clozapine?

It is an antipsychotic drug with no extra pyramidal on endocrinal side effects. It improves negative as well as positive symptoms of schizophrenia. Its main side effect is agranulocytosis. Monitoring of blood count is mandatory. Salivaton, raised blood pressure & convulsions may occur occasionally.

132. What is cheese reaction?

Cheese, beer, wine, pickled meat and fish contain large quantities of tyramin, capable of liberating stored catecholamines. So if patients on monoamine oxidase inhibitor drug consume any of the above mentioned food items, tyramine & other monoamines escape metabolism & tyramine releases stored catecholamines producing hypersensitive crisis & cerebrovascular accident

133. What precautions should be taken during lithium therapy?

Lithium has a very low therapeutic index. Constant monitoring of plasma, lithium concentration is essential. There is no specific antidote for lithium intoxication. Osmotic diuretics, $NaHCO_3$ promotes lithium excretion. Hemodialysis is done when serum lithium level increases.

134. What are uses of sodium valproate?

It is a broad spectrum anti-epileptic, effective against all types of seizures.

135. What is the drug treatment for status epilepticus?

Diazepam 10mg IV over 5 min, Repeated twice more at 15 min. interval. Phenytoin 18-20 mg per kg at more than 50mg per min of seizure, 200mg of phenobarbitone or intubate the patient.

136. What are the adverse effects of levodopa?

Acute effects: Nausea, vomiting, altered sensation, postural hypotension, cardiac arrhythmias, schizophrenia.

Chronic effects: dyskinesia, flocculation's

137. Name drugs used to treat spasticity.

Diazepam, dantroline. They act centrally as muscle relaxant.

Baclofem, act on GABA receptors in the brain.

138. How is morphine metabolised?

It undergoes first pass metabolism. Its half life is 3 – 6 hours. It is metabolized by conjugation and 3 and 6 hydroxyl groups.

139. What are the contra indications for IV barbiturates?

Allergy to barbiturates, severe cardiovascular disease, hypotension, dyspnoea, status asthmaticus, addison's disease, myxedema and hepatic dysfunction.

140. Write the action and nursing consider-

ations of diazepam administrations.

Sedative, they bind to the alpha sub units of GABA a receptors surrounding the chloride channels in the CNS. It is used as anti-convulsants and anesthetics.

Nursing considerations: check for the patient tolerance to the sedative. Check for the arousability of the patient, patient should be on bed rest, assess for physical and psychic dependence and behavioral changes.

141. Mention the therapeuic uses of barbiturates and treatment for barbiturate poisoning.

Antiepileptic, IV anesthesia, Hypnotics, Anticonvulsants, Sedatives.

Treatment: Gastric lavage, hemodialysis, forced diuresis, IV Fluids.

143. Write the pharmacological actions of morphine, what is the specific anti dote in morphin.

It causes analgesia by selectively acting on receptors situated both in the high centers and spinal cord

Naloxone is used as the anti dote for this (0.4-2mg IV, SOS)

144. What are side effects of carbamazepine?

Enzyme induction, drowsiness, dizziness, ataxia, several mental and motor disturbances, water retention, CV side effects, hypersensitivity reaction

145. Name four anti- inflammatory drugs.

- Ibuprofen
- Diclofenac
- Fenofenac
- Indomethacin

146. Name the pure opioid analgesics.

Naloxone, Naltrexone administered orally.

147. Name some mood stabilizers.

- Lithium carbonate
- Carbamazepine
- Sodium valproate

148. List the causes of non-response to neuroleptic therapy.

- Inadequate doses
- Poor patient compliance
- Pharmacokinetic factors
- Persistent and severe psychosocial stress
- Substance abuse

149. List the management of status epilepticus.

- Hospitalisation, adequate ventilation, prevent physical injury, obtain blood samples.
- Establish IV line with NS, 50% glucose and 100 mg thiamin.
- Give anti convulsant and anti-epileptic therapy

150. What are the uses of papaverine?

As a vasodialator (coronary & peripheral) used for intra cavernous injection in erectile impotence. It is a non specific vasodilator

151. List the adverse reaction of paracetamol.

Hepatic and renal toxicity, neutropenia, nephropathy, anemia.

152. What are the uses of caffeine?

- In analgesic mixture
- With ergotamine for the treatment of migraine
- In apnoea in premature infants

153. What are uses of theophylline?

- Asthma & COPD
- Apnoea in premature infants

154. What are the advantages of enalpril over captopril?

- It is more potent
- Longer duration of action through slower onset
- Bind more tightly to converting enzyme & persists longer in the body
- Incidence of rash & taste disturbances

are less frequent

155. In which groups of patients you should not use calcium channel blockers?

- Patients with myocardial inadequacy
- Patients with conduction defects
- Patients with prostate hypertrophy

156. Name the drugs which reduce both preload & after load.

Organic nitrates, ACE inhibitors, sodium nitroprusside, prazosin

157. What are various routes of administration of nitrates?

Sublingual, transdermal, oral, intravenous and especially skin patches.

158. What is the drug of choice for MI?

Morphine sulphate, streptokinase, aspirin, sodium nitroprusside, atropine, beta adrenergic
blockers.

159. What are the drugs used for hypertensive urgencies?

Nifedipine 10mg, clonidine 100 mcg, captopril 25mg, hydralazine 10-20 mg and furosemide.

160. What is the extra cardiac toxicity of digitalis?

GI toxicity- Nausea, vomiting, anorexia. Neurological toxicity- Vertigo, visual disturbances, head ache, neuralgia, pain in face.

161. How is digoxin toxicity treated?

- Stop digoxin and diuretic therapy,
- Atropine to treat AV block
- Monitor potassium level and supraventricular arrhythmias
- Phenytoin

162. What are therapeutic uses of quinidine?

Atrial fibrillation, atrial flutter, paroxysmal atrial and nodal tachycardia and ventricular tachycardia, atrial, ventricular pre mature beats.

163. What are adverse effects of progestines?

Menstrual cycle irregularities, decreased flow, nausea, oesophageal reflexes, acne, edema, breast discomfort, headache, fatigue, depression, liver damage,

164. Name ovulation inducing agents.

Synthetic GnRh, human menopausal and chorionic gonodotropin combination, antiestrogenic combination – cycloferrin

165. What are the contra indications of electrical depolarisation of heart (Cardiversion)?

Digitalis induced arrhythmias, advanced AV block, induced ventricular fibrillation, omit digitalis at least 24 hours before electro version.

166. What is the mechanism of action of nicotinic acid?

It decreases TG and VLDL level rapidly and moderately LDL and cholesterol levels. 20- 80 % fall in TGs and 10-20% in CH occurs. It reduces the production of VLDL by liver and so increases its degradation products.

167. Name the maturation factors.

Maturation factors are vitamin B12 and folic acid. Deficiency of the either vitamins results in defective DNA synthesis and megaloblastic anemia

168. What are metabolic actions of folic acids?

Biosynthesis of pyrinidine, an essential constituent of DNA, inter conversion of certain amino acids, incorporation of format pool. All these reactions are necessary for the synthesis of nucleic acid.

169. What is the pharmacological action of heparin?

Anti coagulant effect. Anti platelet in high

doses, increase bleeding time. Heparin in small doses activates lipoprotein lipase from vessel wall.

170. How is heparin administered? How is heparin therapy monitored?

Sodium or calcium in heparin used either as an IV infusion or as an IV intermittent injection, low dose SC administration for prophylaxis, it is not administered IM.

Therapy is monitored by whole blood clotting time and activated partial thromboplastin time.

171. What is streptokinase?

Streptokinase is a non-enzymatic protein derived from beta hemolytic streptococci. It complexes with plasminogen to liberate plasma.

Uses: Pulmonary embolism, acute MI, venous thromboembolism, deep vein thrombosis.

172. Name the anti platelet drugs.

Aspirin, dazoxiben, blocks thromboxaneA2,

Prostacycline, pentoxyfylline and dipyridamole

173. Mention the drugs used for medical termination of pregnancy.

Methotrexate (25-50mg), tamoxifen 20mg

174. Name agents which can control bleeding.

Agents acting locally-Thrombin, thromboplastin, fibrin, and gel foam, oxidized cellulose, vasoconstictors (1% adrenaline), 20% tannic acid, and glycerin.

175. What is the use of bomocriptine?

It is dopamine agonists. It is used in the following situations - hyperprolactinemia, galactorrhoea syndrome, it stops galactorrhoea and correct amenorrhoea, restores fertility in women and libido potency in man.

176. What are the advantages of radioiodine therapy?

Patient is risk on injury to parathyroid or recurrent laryngeal nerve. Once hyperthyroidism is controlled, cure permanent. It can give in patients not fit for surgery and in patients where oral drugs have failed. Treatment is simple convenient can be given on an out-patient basis and is inexpensive.

177. List the contra indications of calcium channel blockers.

- Tight aortic stenosis
- Severe myocardial depression
- Heart block
- Clinical heart failure
- Unstable angina

178. Name the drugs used in the treatment of CCF.

- Digitalis
- Diuretics
- Vasodilators
- Cardiac stimulants

179. Mention the treatment of shock.

- Adrenaline
- Nor-adrenaline
- Dopamine
- Dobutamine

180. State the anti-platelet drugs.

Prostacycline PGI, inhibitors of TXA2 formation, ADP receptor antagonist, phosphodiesterase inhibitors

181. Classify oral hypoglycemic agents.

Sulfonyl ureas:

First generation - Tolbutamide, chlorpropamide, tolazmide, acetohexamide

Second generation - Glyburide, gylpizide, gliclazide, glymidine

Biguanides: Metformine, phenformin

182. Name some drugs which can be used in pancreatic insulinemia.

- Diazoxide
- Sterptozocin

183. What precautions are to be observed during corticosteroids therapy?

Before starting therapy:

- Inquire about history of peptic ulcer, watch for anemia, diabetics, any infection.
- Take X-ray of chest to rule out TB

During therapy:

- Prescribe the drug with food
- Examine urine periodically for sugar
- Instruct the patient not to stop therapy abruptly
- Keep record of weight and BP
- Increase the dose in infections ion during surgery
- Treat infection with antibiotics
- Taper therapy

184. Classify estrogen preparations?

Natural – Estriol, estrodiol, estro.
Semi synthetic – Ethinyl estrodiol.
Synthetic – steroid and non-steroid.

185. Name some anti-androgens and what are their uses?

Cyproterone acetate, flutamide, ketoconazole, spironolactone, finasteride.

186. Name the drugs used for medical termination of pregnancy.

Methotrexate (25-50)mg, tamoxifen 20 mg.

187. What are the advantages of insulin?

They are purer, neutral and less likely to cause subcutaneous fat atrophy. They are more sable and less antigenic (because of porcine origin)

188. What are the types of insulin?

- Short acting
- Intermediate acting
- Long acting.

189. State the mechanism of action of acarbose.

It binds to carbohydrate binding region of alpha glycosidase enzymes in the brush border of the enterocytes in the jejunum. It inhibits intestinal absorption of carbohydrates.

SOCIOLOGY

INTRODUCTION

Sociology is the study of society. It is the study of human society. It is considered as the social science. All human beings have to interact with other human beings in order to survive.

Study of sociology is considered important as it studies society as a whole. Sociology is important for nurses to maintain physical, psychological and social health of people in the society.

Individual and society

Society is the web of social relationships. Man is a social animal. Community involves any small or large group sharing food, shelter etc. Man is moulded into a social being through the process of socialization. The agents of socialization are family, school, play mates, religion and state.

Culture

Culture has an influence on social role. The culture is acquired and is a social product which fulfills the needs of groups. It is the sum total of ideas and norms of a group and is passed from generation to generation. Culture is usually acquired through enculturation. The culture differs from society to society, so there is diversity. Socialization begins from birth. Culture influences health and disease.

Social groups

Man lives in social groups and these social groups shape the personality of human beings. Groups are most stable and enduring social unit. Groups can be categorized into horizontal, vertical, crowds, class, caste etc. Cooperation is achieved when people work together to achieve the common goal. Conflict is a social process in which individual and groups seek their ends directly challenging the antagonist by violence or threat of violence.

Family and marriage

Family is a biological social unit composed of husband, wife and children. Each family has certain characteristics. A change has been seen in modern family system. Family plays an important role in health and disease.

Social stratification

Social stratification is the hierarchical arrangement and establishment of social categories. Caste is hereditary endogamous group having common name, common traditional occupation, common culture, relatively rigid in matters of mobility. Changes in caste system have been found in last few centuries. Social mobility is the movement of a person from one social status to another.

Social changes

Community

Community is social group having we feeling and living in a given area. Gram panchayat is a basic unit and executive organ of gram sabha. Community can be urban and rural community.

Social change

Social change is the difference in the social phenomenon over a period of time. Social change is a continuous process as the change in population, technology, values and ideologies keep on occurring. Social change differs from society to society and is influenced by various factors. Nurse acts as a change agent, who seeks to fully understand the individual and community and uses this knowledge to create focused goals to achieve the needed change.

Social control

Social control is an influence which is exercised by society for the promotion of welfare of group as a whole. It is considered important as it controls the member's behavior in society and is essential for maintaining continuity and uniformity in society.

Social problems

Social disorganization occurs when various parts of society fail to adjust themselves to changing conditions. Social problems are threat to society which need to be eliminated. A number of social problems occur in society which are categorized into economic, biological, bio psychological and cultural.

Nurses play an important role in controlling social problems. She assess the poverty level of people while doing home visits. She makes them aware of various means of economic growth of family and counsels them. She also assesses overall social problems and does activities to reduce health problems.

References

1. Kumari N. (2010). **A Textbook of Sociology**, 3rd ed. Vikas.
2. Purushothama GS. (2010). **Nursing Sociology**. 1st ed. Jaypee.

Test Series

1. **What is sociology?**
The word sociology is derived from the latin word 'societus' meaning 'society' and Greek word 'logos' meaning 'study or science'.
"Sociology is the study of human interaction and interrelation of their condition and consequences"
"Sociology is the science of society or of social phenomena"
2. **What are the characteristics of sociology?**
The characteristics are:
Social, categorical, pure, abstract, generalizing, rational, empirical and general.
3. **What are the two aspects of formal school of sociology?**
   - Form
   - Content
4. **What are the main principles of formal school of sociology?**
   - It does not study the things or factors connected with the social phenomena
   - Since every science has a special scope or a field of specialization, this is true of sociology as well.
5. **What are the weaknesses of formal school of sociology?**
   - Unpractical
   - The concept of form and content and unpractical classification
   - Limitation of the scope of the study.
6. **Write about the criticism of formalistic school.**
   - It has narrowed the scope of sociology
   - Abstract forms separated from concrete relations cannot be studied
   - The conception of pure sociology is impractical
   - Sociology alone does not study social relationships
7. **What are the principles of synthetic school of sociology?**
   - Organic structure of the society
   - Different social sciences study different aspects of the society.
8. **What are the chief exponents of the synthetic school?**
Durkheim, Hob house, Ginsberg and Sorokin.
9. **What is the importance of sociology?**
Helpful in social reconstruction
Useful in solution of various social problems
Helpful in planning and emotional integration Necessary for labour welfare
10. **Specify the objectives of sociology.**
To introduce sociology knowledge to nurses, understanding a wide range of under graduate & post graduate courses

To promote an inquisitive & reflective mode of conducting nursing work

11. Name the factors involved in the process of socialization.

Imitation, suggestion, identification and language

12. Name the agencies of socialization.

The family, the school, the playmates or friends, the church and the state.

13. Define health.

Health is defined as the state of complete physical, mental and social well being and not merely the absence of disease or infirmity.

14. Name the social factors influencing health status.

Housing, occupation, financial and social status, climate, geography, nutrition, norms and roles of the society in which the individual lives, personal characteristics of the individual which include age, sex, genetic makeup, intellect and personality, personal habits behavioural characteristics & medical history.

15. What is individualization?

Individualization is the process in which man comes to know himself, acquire the sense of inner responsibility.

16. What are aspects of individualization?

Manheim has distinguished four main aspects of individualization. These are:

- Individualization as a process of learning different from other people
- Individualization through objects
- Individualization on the level of new forms of self regarding attitudes
- Individualization as a kind of deepening into ourselves which implies receiving into our experience of ourselves and sublimating the individualizing forces around and within us.

17. What are the elements of socialization?

- The physical and psychological heritage of the individual
- Environment in which he is born.
- Culture in which he lives..

18. List down some factors promoting health or illness.

- Lack of information or education on health care.
- Lack of transport facilities to enable contact with doctors, hospitals.
- Difficult access to building
- Lack of support.
- Limited protection by legislation.
- Lack of ones or limited access to financial support.

19. Name some methods to improve social consciousness about health.

- Teaching about the personal hygiene by parents to their children.
- Teachers must educate students about preventive methods of common sickness and injuries.
- The prime duty of a nurse is to give health education to public, primary level of preventive measures to control communicable and infective diseases.

20. What is society?

Society is the complex of organized associations and institutions with a community. Society is a web of social relationship.

21. What is socialization in rehabilitation of patients?

Rehabilitation is to bring back the physically disable or delinquent into normal life by special treatment. Rehabilitation is a process of socialization of assisting individuals with handicapped to realize particular goals physically, mentally, socially, economically.

22. Name the two theories concerned with the nature of society?

- The social contract theory.
- The organism theory

23. Difference society and community.

Society	Community
Rural society	Urban society
- Less mobile - Homogenous - Dominated by primary relations - Ppeople are simple, hospitable, frank and generous.	- Mmore mobile -Heterogenous - Dominated by secondary relations - People are artificial, narrow minded and selfish.
- Abstract - More than one community - Web of social relationship - Definite geographic area is not an essential aspect.	- Concrete - Smaller than Society. - Some degree of we feeling - Definite locality or geographic area.

24. Define culture.

Culture is that complex whole which includes knowledge, belief, art, morals, law, custom, and any other capabilities acquired by man as a member of society.

25. What are the elements of culture?

- Culture is a learned behaviour of pattern
- Culture is a pattern of living, a design for living
- Culture is passed from generation to generation.

26. What are characteristics of culture?

- Culture is based on some ideals and norms of behaviour and each member has to follow them.
- It is learned by each person in the course of his development in a particular situation.
- Language is the chief vehicle of culture.
- Culture is always linked with past experiences and keeps on developing as it passes from generation to generation.

27. Name the components of culture.

- **Cultural traits**-Learned pattern of behaviour
- **Culture pattern**-Forms traits and complexes become related to each other in functional roles.
- **Culture complex**-Larger cluster of traits.

28. What are the cultural traits giving rise to cultural pattern?

- Speech and language
- Material traits like food habits, shelter, dress, utensils, weapons
- Art
- Religious practices
- Property
- Government

29. Write about the evolution of culture.

The basic process valid in cultural development is discovery and invention. All cultural traits, material as well as non material have been invented at sometime and in some place by some person, but no single invention contributes to the development of culture. It is only an addition to what already exists.

30. Name the reason for cultural variability.

- Historical accidents
- Geographical environment
- Mobility of human organism

- Invention and discoveries
- Individual peculiarities or personal eccentricities
- Change in the modes of production
- Dominant cultural themes

31. Write about diversity and uniformity of culture.

Diversity of culture

- The do's and don'ts of some societies are the don'ts and do's of other society.
- One culture insists about a woman marrying certain relative but other culture forbid it.
- The young generation differs greatly in terms of own manners, values and commitment.

Uniformity

Every culture found murder and lying, need of marriage and family, but different cultures have different ideas about each above.

32. What are the functions of culture?

In Individual

- Culture makes a man, a human being
- Culture provides solutions for complicated situations
- Culture provides traditional interpretations to certain situations

In Group

- Culture keeps social relationships intact.
- Culture broadens the vision of the individual.
- Culture creates new needs.

33. Define cultural diffusion.

It is the process by which the cultural traits invented are discovered in one society and are spread directly to another society.

34. Write the demographic process.

- Fertility
- Mortality
- Marriage
- Migration
- Social mobility

35. What are social problems of population explosion?

- Drug abuse
- Alcoholism
- Corruption
- Terrorism
- Poverty
- Unemployment
- Family disorganization
- Sexual deviance
- Organized crimes

36. Define social problems.

"A condition which is defined by a considerable number of persons as a deviation from social norms which they cherish.

- Fuller And Myres

37. What are the cultural basis of social problems?

- Widow's marriage
- Child marriage
- Restriction on inter cost marriages
- Problems of Devadasi
- Smoking of marijuana

38. What are the consequence of population changes in agrarian countries?

- Rising poverty and retards development
- Youth unemployment and political instability
- Pressure on land and migration

39. What are the consequence of population change in the industrialized countries?

- The costs of goods and services become costly
- Over urbanization
- Environmental degradation
- Population growth, degrades the quality of life

- Problems of migration

40. List down the causes of population growth in India.

- Peaceful conditions and achievements in medical science and elimination of infectious disease
- Widening gap between birth and death rate
- Universal and low age at marriage
- High illiteracy and poverty
- Development in agriculture and industry
- The persistency of joint family system
- Tropical climatic condition
- Religious attitude towards family planning

41 What are the evil effects of population explosion?

- Pressure on land
- Shortage of food
- Poor levels of health
- Housing shortage
- Unemployment and economic losses

42. What are the curative plans of population control?

- Rapid industrialization
- Improvement in agriculture
- Planned migration

43. What are the preventive plans of population control?

- Rise in the age at marriage
- Increasing urbanization and industrialization
- Compulsory education
- Social security measures
- Planned parenthood
- Change in tax structure for procreation

44. Define family.

"It is the biological social unit, which is composed of husband, wife and children"

OR

"More or less durable association of husband and wife with or without child or of man and women with children"

45. What are the concepts of family?

- Biological concept
- Psychological concept
- Economical concept
- Sociological concept

46. State the characteristics of family.

- Making permanent relationship between husband and wife through sexual relationship
- A form of mutual relationship established and maintained
- Financial provision shared by two members of a group to fulfill economic needs
- Common habitation
- University
- It is for the mature agency of socialization, family members have certain responsibilities duties and obligations etc
- It may be permanent or temporary in nature
- The family is guarded both by social taboos and legal regulations

47. Which system theory mainly focuses on family concept?

System theory is focused on internal and external relationship and dynamics.So this concept is more applicable for community health nursing.

48. What is patriarchal family?

The father is the most powerful in the family. Such a family is called patriarchal family

49. What is matriarchal family?

Mother plays a dominant role in a family.

Such a family is called a matriarchal family

50. What is matrilocal?

The husband lives in the wife's home

51. What is patrilocal?

The wife lives in the husband's home

52. What is changing residence?

Husband and wife alternatively change their residence is called changing residence

53. Define polygamy.

One marries many women and lives in a family with all of them or with each of them alternatively

54. Define monogamous.

One man marry only one women and establish a family is called monogamous

55. Define metronymic.

Family is the named after the mother

56. What is patronymic?

Family is named after the father

57. What is nuclear family?

This is the elementary family or married couple and their unmarried children

58. Define joint family.

The joint family is a mode of combining smaller family in to lager family, units through the extension of three or more generations including at least grandparents, parents and children

59. What is extended family?

Husband, wife, children and other dependents like brother, sister stay together.

60. What are the functions of the family?

- Sexual gratification
- Primary socialization of individual occurs
- Social and mental stress are overcome
- Social and economic support is obtained
- Social interaction brings about new knowledge
- Each members has a role to play and job responsibility
- Provision of food, education, housing, clothing which are necessary to existence of human life

61. What are the basic needs of a family?

Family is a vital social institution, fundamental units of society.

The basic needs of the family are started below

- **Physical**: Food, safe water, clothing, safe environment, shelter, safe disposal of water
- **Biological**: Free from communicable diseases, control of insects and rodents
- **Psychological**: Happy home, adequate medical care, safe working environment, psycho-social security

62. What is the importance of family?

- Face to face contact of members will be established
- Intimate long lasting relationship are developed
- It develops character of the members in the family and the society
- Maintain social organization teaches accepted way of behavior
- Individual acquires healthy characteristics like honesty, sympathy responsibility
- Family members help for individual personality
- It is a conveyance of tradition
- Family encourages blossom of interest in different areas like education, helps in intellectual development always.

63. What are the problems of family?

- Health problems: Diarrhea, STD, skin infection, malignancy

- Environmental problems: Atmospheric pollution (air, water pollution), road accidents
- Economic problems: Poverty
- Social problems: Alcoholism, drug abuse, prostitution
- Psychological problem: Anxiety, stress, suicides.

64. What are the reasons for changing Indian family system?

Changes are mainly due to

- Varied social interaction
- Progressive urbanization
- Civilization

65. What are the changes in Indian family?

- Loosening of social regulation
- Indian women's behaves like western culture
- Faces difficulty in reproductive and child health period
- Deteriorating kingship in the family
- Diverse rate is increasing
- There is considerable diversity in family norms

66. What are the changes in modern family?

- Decreased control on marriage contract
- Changes in relationship of man and women
- Laxity in sex relationship
- Mostly child rearing is by contract workers
- Re-marriages
- Decline of patriarchal authority
- Female partner head of the family in many cases
- Economic independence
- Decline of religious control
- Decreasing family values

67. What are the reasons for changes in modern family?

Accessibility and availability of social and economic sanctions

68. Define marriage.

Marriage is a socially approved relation which allows sexual relationship between two individuals of opposite sex. According to Malinowski, "Marriage is a contract for the production and maintenance of children". Marriage forms basis of a procreation with an expectation that married couples will produce and bring up children.

69. What is the importance of marriage?

- It insists the couple to establish family by procreation
- Regulation of sex life and sex relation of the individual
- Put restrictions on the pre-marital and extra-marital sex relations
- Marriage helps intellectual co-operations among both of them
- Minimizes the social distance between groups and strengthens their sociality

70. What are types of marriage?

- Monogamy
- Endogamy
- Polygamy/exogamy
- Polyandry
- Matriarchal marriage
- Consanguineous marriage
- Patriarchal marriage

71. What is polyandry?

One women having many husbands is called polyandry

72. What is exogamy?

Marrying with outside two groups or caste

73. What is group marriage?

Marriage are held in a common place by a group of brides and bride grooms.

74. What are the problems of marriage in India?

- Dowry system
- Lack of trust
- Sex laxity
- Sexual heterogeneity
- Decline of family control, moral values
- Inferior and superior complexes
- Impact of western family system

75. What are common legislations related to marriage?

The laws enacted in India related to marriage are

- Age at marriage (18 to 21)
- Number of spouses in marriage
- Field of male selection
- Breaking of marriage
- Re-marriage
- Dowry

76. List Marriage Acts.

It means a law made by a government about marriage

- Prevention of Sati Act (1829)
- Hindu Widow Re-marriage Act (1856)
- The Civil for Special Marriage Act (1872)
- The Hindu marriage Act (1955)
- Dowry Prohibition Act (1961)
- Child Marriage Restraint Sct (CMRA) (1929

77. Define social stratification.

- Stratification is a process by which individuals and groups are ranked in a more or less enduring hierarchy of status - Ogburn & Nimkoff
- Social stratification is a horizontal division of society into higher and lower social units - Raymond and Murry
- Social stratification is a division of society into permanent categories linked with each other by the relationship of superiority and subordination.

78. Mention the types of social stratification.

- Caste Stratification-(Brahmin, Kshatrya, Vaishya, Shudra)
- Racial Stratification
- Class Stratification

79. Enlist the characteristics of social stratification.

It is universal in nature

- It is an ancient phenomenon
- It is social
- Stratification is found in different forms
- It is consequential

80. Define caste.

A collection of families or group of families bearing a common name, claiming common dissect from a mythical ancestor human or divine professing to follow the same hereditary calling and regarded by those who are competent to give an opinion as forming a single homogenous

81. What are the legislation, which integrate the caste system in India?

- The Caste Disabilities Removal Act of 1850
- The special marriage act of 1872
- The Hindu Widow Remarriage Act 1856

82. List down the merits of caste system and trade unions.

- Spirit of co-operation
- Defines economic pursuits
- Racial purity
- Influences intellectual make up
- Integration of the country
- Provides for varies countries in the society
- Cultural diffusion
- Separation of social from political life

83. What are de-merits of caste system?

Deprives mobility of labour.
Untouchability
Solidarity retarded
Wrong men in occupation
Obstacle to national unity
Obstacle to social progress
Undemocratic

84. Point out theories of the origin of caste system.

Racial theory
Political theory
Occupational theory
Traditional theory
Guild theory
Religious theory
Evolutionary theory

85. Write the traditional features of caste.

Caste as a segmental division of society
Caste panchayats
Caste councils

86. Write the features which impact caste in India today.

- Changes in land reforms and political democracy
- Development of caste for occupation
- Modern education
- Industrialization
- Urbanization
- Westernization
- Religious conversions
- Transport and communication
- Social legislation
- Equal status to women

87. What are the changes in the role of caste system?

- Elections based on caste system
- Constitutional provision for scheduled caste, scheduled tribes & other backward classes
- Impact of modern education
- Increase of caste consciousness
- Increase in caste conflicts

88. Write reasons for change in caste system?

- Uniform legal system
- Impact of modern education
- Industrialization, urbanization, westernization
- Influence of modern transport and communication system
- Freedom from struggle and establishment of democracy
- Rise of non-Brahmin movement

89. What are factors that lead to the growth of cities?

- Surplus resources
- Industrialization
- Commercialization
- Development of transport and communication
- Economic pull of city
- Educational and recreational facilities

90. Mention the factors which facilitate the growth of caste system in India.

- The geographic isolation
- The influence of religion
- The existence of many races
- The rural social structure
- The unwillingness of rulers
- Lack of education
- Hereditary occupations

91. Define social class.

- A social class are the aggregate persons having essentially the same status in a given society
- Ogburn and Nimkoff
- A social class is a culturally defined group that is accorded a particular position or a status within the population as a whole

92. List the characteristics of social class.

- Class is universal.
- Class is a distinct status group
- Class is an opened group
- Class is an opened system
- Classification of social classes
- Criterion of classes

93. Mention the classification of social class.

- The upper-upper class
- The lower-upper class
- The upper-middle class
- The lower-middle class
- The upper-lower class
- The lower-lower class

94. What is class consciousness?

It is the inner aspect of class. It consist of the realization of a similarity of an attitude and behavior with members of other classes

95. Mention the conditions that promote class consciousness.

- Ease and amount of mobility
- Rivalry and conflict
- Growth of common tradition

96. Define social mobility.

Social mobility refers to the moments of individuals and groups between different socio- economic positions

97. What are the types of social mobility?

Horizontal mobility: It refers to the movement of the person from one social position to another of the same rank Vertical mobility: A man moving from one job to another but at much the same levels of the prestige or income is known as horizontal mobility .

98. What is vertical mobility?

It refers to the movement of the person from one social to another of different rank. It may involve moving upward (job of higher rank) or downward job of lower rank. Down ward mobility is less common than upward.

99. Differentiate class and caste.

S.No	Caste	Class
1.	Determined by birth	Determined on the economic status
2.	Unchangeable	Changeable
3.	Closed system	Open system
4.	Restrictions on food and social intercourse	No restrictions
5.	There is endogamy	No endogamy
6.	Strong consciousness of caste	There is class consciousness
7.	Complexity	Simplicity
8.	Conservative	Progressive

100. What is the inter-generational mobility?

When changes occurs from one generation to another it is known as intergenerational mobility. It involves a changes in social positions. E.g:.The bus conductor whose father was an engineer is an example of intergeneration mobility

A film star whose father is a farmer illustrates upwards intergenerational mobility.

101. What is intra-generational mobility?

When mobility occurs in one generation itself is called intra generational carrier mobility. It involves changes in social position within his or her life.

A man who enters as a school teacher and eventually became inspector of school of district is an example of intra-generational upward mobility

102. What is structural /stratum mobility?

- It refers to the vertical movement of a specific group, class or occupation relative to others in the stratification system.
- For example, modern information technologies has made machines and computer technicians more important in society
- They are receiving more respect previously reserved for lawyers and scientists.

103. Define status?

It is defined as a social position in a group or a social system such as female, student, teacher, child, mother, father, etc.

104. List down the types of status.

- Ascribed status: Which are given to as birth (age, sex, kinship, rate, caste) are known as ascribed status
- Achieved status: Any social position held by an individual as a result of his or her personal accomplishment, through his own efforts

105. Differentiate status and role.

S.No	Status	Role
1	Status is a structural phenomenon	Role is the behavior phenomenon
2	Status depends upon social structure	Role depends upon the personality and capability of individuals

106. Define role.

A role is a set of socially expected and approved behavior pattern consisting of both duties and privileges associated particular position in a group.

107. Define role conflict.

Role conflict is a situation in which a person is expected to play two incompatible roles.

108. How will you minimize or reduce the effects of role conflict?

- Choose the role which is more important
- Leave one of the conflicting statuses, for e.g., a person may quit job if it interferes
- Too much with his parenting responsibilities
- Role distance-some disclaimful detachment of the performance from the role he is performing

109. What are types of role differentiation?

- Based on sex – (male, female)
- Based on age –(infancy to old age)
- Based on occupation-(occupation ranking, occupation and prestige income costumes)

110. What are the dimensions of the role?

- Expressive roles and role requiring restrains
- Role based on ascribed status and achieved status
- More focused and more diffused role
- General and specific role
- Self oriented and public oriented roles

111. Define race.

A race is a large biological human grouping with a number of distinctive inherited characteristic which vary within a certain range.

112. List down the characteristics of different race .

Texture and color of hair:

- Leiotrichy (soft strait hair) as of Mongolian, Chinese, Korean etc.
- Cymotrichy (smooth and curly hair) India, western Europe, Australia
- Ulotrichy (thick curly hair) as negroes

Structure of the head:

Which is classified according to the ratio of

length and width

- Doliococephalic
- Mesocophalic
- Brachycephalic

Facial characteristic : Such as nosal form, lab form, eyelid, check chin, ears, jawer.

Nosal forms has 3 types

1) Leptorrhine (thin)
2) Mesorrhine (medium)
3) Platyrhine

- The composition of the skin
- Color of the skin
- Leukoderma as Cancasion
- Xanthoderma as Mongolian
- Melanoderma as Negroes

Based on the principal diameter of the body, chest diameter

- Define racial pre-judice –
- Tall stature (170cm or 5ft 7 inches)
- Above average stature (160cm below 5 feet 5 inches)

Blood group

There are 4 types of blood groups A, B, AB, and O.

113. Define pre-judice.

Pre-judice is an attitude that predisposes a person to think, perceive, feel and act in favorable or unfavorable ways towards the group or its individual members

Race prejudice is the result of social indoctrination and socialization, which is threatening to world peace

114. What are the causes of racial prejudice?

- Economic advantage
- Political advantage
- Ethnocentrism
- Compensation for frustration
- Lack of proper education

115. List races in India.

- Pre-Dravidian type – Tribes of hills and tribes
- The Dravidian type – Indo-Gangetic valley
- Indo-aryan type found in Punjab, Kashmir and Rajasthan
- Arya-dravidan type found in Gangetic valley
- Mongoloid type found in Assam
- Mongoloid Dravidian type in West Bengal and Orissa

116. Define social consciousness.

Social consciousness is the awareness of the similarity of social chances, arising of a similarity of a notion about similarity of interest, the growth of an emotional tie connected with this similarity of experiences and of a common striving towards a common social goal.-Mannheim

117. Define urbanization.

The process of urbanization takes places due to the mobility of the people from rural to urban areas, mainly in search of employment, marriage of girl, education of children.

It is the one of the strongest factors in the transmission of the Indian society.

118. What is social movement?

Social movement defined as "a collectively acting with some continuity promote or resist a change in the society or group of which it is a part.

119. What are factors influencing migration ?

- Poverty due to natural calamities
- Unemployment and lure for higher income
- Urban thrill and urban life
- Large family and small property
- Seasonal employment
- No land for cultivation

120. Define community.

Community is defined as an area marked by the sentiment of common living, (a) a group of people (b) with in a geographic area (c) with a common culture and a social system (d) whose members are conscious of their unity and (e) who can act collectively in an organized manner.

121. Name the two basic elements in the concept of community.

- The community as locality (geographic area)
- The community as sentiment (sentiment of unity)

122. What is ecology?

Ecology is a branch of biology. It is the study of relations between organisms and their environment

123. What is human ecology?

It means the study of inter relationship with their physical environments. Human ecology is the study of how people and institutions are located in space and how do they adjust themselves to their environments. Human ecology includes the study of community and population.

124. Classify communities.

- Neighbourhood
- Village
- City
- Religion and
- World Community

125. State the meaning of neighborhood.

The neighborhood is the first community with which the child comes into contact. It is a loose integration of several family groups

126. Who are migratory communities?

The earliest human communities were perhaps the loosely organised aggregations of a few families who carried on mutually interdependent activities in gathering food and defending themselves against their enemies. These primitive bands were migratory communities.

127. When human communities became more stationary?

With the development of agriculture and the consequent stabilization of the source of food, The people began to lead a settled life.

128. What is the oldest permanent community of man?

The village is the oldest permanent community of man.

129. What are the stages of evolution of village community?

(i) Primitive village community
(ii) Medieval village community
(iii) Modern village community

130. Enlist the features of village community.

Community consciousness-Faith in religion
Role of neighborhood-Simplicity
Joint family

131. List down the factors influencing growth of village.

Topographical factors- land, water, climate
Economic factors-condition of agriculture, rural economy, cottage industries.
Social factors – peace, security, cooperation etc.

132. How many villages are there in India?

There are 5,75,721 Villages in India

133. What are the characteristics of Indian villages?

The characteristics of Indian villages includes:

Isolation and self sufficiency
Peace and simplicity
Conservatism
Poverty and illiteracy

Local self government

134. What is conservatism?

The inhabitants of the village are strongly attached to old customs and traditions. Their outlook is primarily conservative and they accept changes with extreme reluctance.

135. Why All India Kisan Sammelan has been formed ?

It has been formed for rural reconstruction,to focus the attention of the government on the problems of peasantry class.

136. What is the function of ministry of rural development?

It has been formed at the center to look after the over all task of rural development and coordinate the different schemes in this direction.

137. Enlist the schemes of rural development.

- Small Farmers Development Project (SFDP)
- Marginal Farmers and Agricultural Laborers Project (MFAL)
- Drought Prone Aareas Program (DPAP)
- Integrated Rural Development Program (IRDP)
- Applied Nutrition Programme (ANP)
- Jawahar Rozgar Yojana Programme. (JRYP)

138. When panchayat raj was made effective.

The 73rd amendment act, 1993 has sought to make the Panchayat raj system more effective and role playing in the field of rural development.

139. List some of the development that took place in rural community.

- Introduction of labour sewing machinery has shortened farm hours
- Link roads are constructed
- Electricity provided
- Sanitary conditions improved
- Health facilities provided.

140. Define urban community.

The census report have defined

(i) Those which have a local authority like municipality cantonment board, notified area committees,

(ii) All other places which satisfy the requirements of a minimum population of 5,000 at least 75% of the male working population engaged in non agricultural pursuits and a density of population of at least 900 persons per sq km.

141. Classify cities.

- Production centers, such as Jamshedpur for iron and steel
- Centers of trade and commerce, example: New York
- Political capitals for instance, New Delhi
- Cultural centers like Oxford
- Resort cities like Srinagar, Simla
- Diversified cities

142. When did the first city appear?

The first cities seem to have appeared sometime between 6000 and 5000 BC. These cities were however small and hard to distinguish from towns. By 3000 BC, there were in existence what may be called true cities.

143. What is a region?

A region is a large area where there are a good many resemblances among the inhabitants. A region is defined as an area within which the people and the different constituent communities are conspicuously more inter dependent than they are with people of other areas

144. What is a physical region?
A physical region is one which is demarcated by geographical factors. A large river valley surrounded by a mountain is a well-known type of physical region.

145. State the meaning of a metropolitan region.
A metropolitan region is a large city with its suburbs and all the surrounding area whose trading activities are carried on in the city.

146. What is a sectional region?
A sectional region is one in which a particular set of folk ways prevail.

147. State meaning of administrative region.
An administrative region is governed by political boundaries determined by convenience or by accident or by political planning.

148. What are the regions in India?
(i) **Northern zone** – Jammu Kashmir, New Delhi.
(ii) **Western zone** – Maharashtra, Gujarat.
(iii) **Southern zone** – Madras, Mysore, Kerala
(iv) **Eastern zone** – Assam, Orissa.

149. What is nation?
A nation is a historical and sociological phenomenon and that the nation evolved out of the amalgam of various racial and kinship groups after the break- up of the slaving –owning and feudal societies.

150. What is change?
The word 'change' denotes a difference in anything observed over some period of time.

151. State the meaning of social change.
Social change means observable differences in any social phenomena over any period of time.

152. Define social change.
According to jones, `social change' is a term used to describe variation in or modification of, any aspect of social processes, social patterns, social interaction or social organization.

153. What are excluded from social change.
Social change does not refer to all the changes going on in the society. The changes in art, language, technology, philosophy etc. may not be included in the term 'social change'.

154. What are social relationship?
Social relationships are social processes, social patterns, and social interactions.

155. Why social changes are a universal phenomenon?
It occurs in all societies. No society remains completely static. This is true of all societies, primitive as well as civilized.

156. Why social change is a community change?
Social change does not refer to the change in the life of an individual or the life pattern of several individuals. It is a change which occurs in the life of the entire community.

157. Is the speed of social change uniform?
No, while social change occurs in all society, its speed is not uniform in every society. It is faster in urban areas than in rural areas.

158. What affects the speed of social change?
Nature and speed of social changes is affected by and related to time factor. Before 1917 there was a less industrialization in India, therefore the speed of social change after 1917 is faster than before.

159. Why social change occurs as an essential law?
Changes is a law of nature. Social change also is natural. It may occur either in the

natural course or as planned effort because of our need keep on changing. To satisfy our desire for change and our changing needs social change becomes a necessity.

160. Is definite prediction of social change possible?

No, it is difficult to make any prediction about the exact forms of social change.

161. Why social change shows chain reaction sequence?

Social change is shows chain reaction sequence because a society`s pattern of living is a dynamic system of inter related parts.

162. Why social change results from the interaction of number of factors?

Social phenomena or mutually interdependent. None stand out has isolated forces that bring about change of themselves. Modification of one part influences the other parts and this influences the rest, until the whole is involved.

163. What are the four ages according to Indian mythology? ?

Man has passed through four ages – Satyug, Treata, Dwapur and Kaliyug.

164. What is the life cycle of a society?

Society has predetermined life cycle and has birth, growth, maturity and decline.

165. What is theory of deterioration?

Deterioration began to take place with the result that man reached an age of comparative degeneration.The satyug was the best age in which man was honest, truthful and perfectly happy, thereafter degeneration began to take place.

166. What is cyclic theory?

Society after passing through all the stages, returns to the original stage, where the cycle begins again. Satyug will again start after kaliyug is over.

167. What is theory of biological cycle?

Western civilization is doomed to extinction because of the constant infiltration of foreign inferior elements and their increasing control over it. It will decline soon and all ancient civilization will start beginning.

168. What was propounded by Vilfredo Pareto?

Wilfredo Pareto propounded the theory that societies pass through the periods of political vigor and decline which repeat themselves in cyclical fashion.

169. Define social organization.

It can be defined as "state of being a condition in which the various institutions in a society are functioning in accordance with their recognized or implied purposes".

170. Enlist the three elements of social organizations.

- Society
- Culture
- Personality

Also, social organization emphasizes coordination of social relationship

- a goal
- preparedness to accept ones role and status
- norms and mores
- sanction

171. Enlist the four fundamental rights of individuals.

- Right to equality
- Right of freedom
- Right towards culture and education
- Right of property

172. Define voluntary organization.

According to Michall Banton, "voluntary organization is a group of people organized for the pursuit of one interest or of several interest common".

173. State the meaning of voluntary association.

Voluntary association is a group of persons organized on the basis of voluntary membership without state control for the furtherance of some common interest of its members.

174. List down the four characteristics of voluntary association.

- It has own administrative structure and a duly constitute management
- It has governed by its own members on democratic principle without any external control
- It has definite objective and purposes and programmes for their fulfillment and achievement
- It collects and save fund for its activities in the form of contribution or subscription from the members of local community and aboard.

175. Define social system.

- Social system is an orderly and symptomatic arrangement of social interactions
- It is a network of interactive relationships
- It is defined as a "plurality of individuals interacting with each other according to shared cultural norms and meanings
- Social system is an organization as it is an elderly and systematic arrangements of parts.

176. Mention four important features of social system.

- Basement of social system is social interaction
- The interaction process should carry some meaning
- The part of social system are integrated
- Social system has a definite environment

177. Enlist four basic elements of social system.

- Belief and knowledge
- Sentiments
- Norms
- Status and role

178. Enlist the Morgan's classification of social system.

- Hunting social system
- Agricultural social system
- Industrial social system
- Pastoral social system

179. Enlist the Sorokins classification of social system.

- Sensate
- Ideational
- Idealistic

180. Name Darkheims social system.

- Mechanic social system
- Organic social system

181. Define social role.

According to Lundberg "social role is a pattern of behavior expected of an individual in certain group or situation".

182. List different types of social role.

- Achievement role
- Recruitment role
- Occupational role

183. What are the three pre-requisites of social system?

- Biological pre-requisites
- Functional pre-requisites
- Cultural pre-requisites

184. List down three functional pre-requisites.

- Obedience to social norms

- Mechanism of social control
- Interest towards positive action

185. What are the three main culture pre-requisites?
- Language
- Symbol
- System of communication

186. What are mechanisms of social system?
- Mechanism of socialization
- Mechanism of social control

187. What is status?

According to Ogburn and Nimkoff "status represents the position of individual in the group."

188. Enlist two types of status.
- Ascribed status
- Achieved status

189. What is ascribed status?

It is not based on one's own effort, his capabilities and his abilities. It is based on one's caste, family background etc.

190. What are the four factors that determine ascribed status?
- Age
- Sex
- Caste
- race

191. What is achieved status?

An individual is achieving his status by his own effort and capabilities.

Eg: an individual's position in an institution.

192. What are the four determinatives of achieved status?
- Education
- Occupation
- Marriage
- Wealth

193. What are the types of disorganization?
- Personal or individual disorganization
- Crime, prostitution and drug addiction
- Family disorganization
- Divorce, separation, broken homes
- Community disorganization
- Poverty, beggary, unemployment-Elliot

194. What are the differences between the role and status?

Role	Status
Roles are properly established on the needs of society.	Status is established based on social aspiration and ambition
Roles are different from one individual to another.	Status represents only a part of social setup.

195. What are the types of social institutions?
- Family
- Education
- Religion
- Economic
- State

196. What are the types of disorganization?
- Personal or individual disorganization
- Crime, prostitution and drug addiction
- Family disorganization
- Divorce, separation, broken homes
- Community disorganization
- Poverty, beggary, unemployment-Elliot

196. Point out the causes of personal disorganization.
- Biological factors (physical, mental)
- Environmental factor (economic stress
- Loss of security (wealth)
- Crisis in life (sudden shock, accident, death, loss of job)

197. List the causes of social disorganization
- Psychological factors-Communication and the problems of the attitude.
- Cultural lag-Adopting western technology
- Physical or geographic factors-Storms, cyclones, floods
- Biological factors-Related to environmental in terms of regions and neigh-

borhood. e.g:. housing, overcrowding

- Social problems-Financial revolution
- Degeneration of values-Art, science, philosophy etc …
- Disintegration and confusion of roles
- Political sub-ordination

198. What are the characteristics of social disorganization?

- Conflicts of mores and of institutions
- Transfer of functions from one group to another
- Individuation and individualistic tendencies
- Inconsistency between expectations and achievements
- Inconsistency between status and rule

199. What are the remedial measures to face the social disorganization?

- Proper and comprehensive social and economic planning and policies
- Proper implementation of plans and policies
- Organized social welfare activities
- Appropriate steps to rehabilitate and reform the beggars, criminals, juvenile delinquencies, prostitutes, mentally and physically handicapped, the aged, and the diseased persons
- To mobilize public opinion

200. Define poverty.

Poverty is the insufficient of those thing as which are requisite for an individual to maintain himself and those dependent upon him in health and vigor-Goddard,J.G

201. Mention the types of poverty.

- Absolute poverty
- Relative poverty

202. List down the causes of poverty.

- Landlessness
- Sickness
- Illiteracy and ignorance
- Extravagancy
- Unhealthy habits
- Natural calamities
- Unemployment
- overpopulation
- Lack of supporting industries, poor marketing industries system
- Lack of facilities for poor transportation

203. What are remedial measures for poverty?

- The five year plans
- Nationalization
- 20 point programme
- IRDP, NREP JRY
- Legislation to prevent poverty
- Establishment of protective homes
- Provision of workhouses
- Comprehensive social security measures
- Mobilizing public opinion
- Scheme to collect donation

204. Expand IRDP, NREP, RLEP, TRYSEM.

- IRDP-Integrated Rural Development Programme
- NREP – National Rural Employment Programme
- RLEP – Rural Landless Employment Guarantee Programme
- TRYSEM –Training Rural Youth For Self Employment

205. Definition of social problems.

- It is a condition which is defined by a considerable number of person as a deviation from social norms which they cherish

206. List down social problems in India.

- Population explosion
- Unemployment
- Food shortage
- Ill health

- Low standard of living
- Poverty
- Malnutrition
- Frustration
- Suicide
- Family disorganization
- Untouchability
- Child marriage
- Prostitution
- Dowry
- Child labor
- Juvenile delinquency

207. Mention the causes of population explosion in India.

- Peaceful conditions and achievements in medical sciences
- Widening gap between birth and death rate
- Universal and low age at marriage
- High illiteracy and poverty
- Development in agriculture and industries
- The persisting of joint family system
- Tropical climatic conditions
- Religious attitude towards family planning

208. List down the evil effects of population explosion.

- Pressure on land
- Shortage of food
- Poor levels of health
- Housing shortage
- Unemployment and economic losses

209. How can we overcome population?

Creative plans or increasing production

- Rapid industrialization
- Improvements in agriculture
- Planned migration

Preventing plans for population control

- Rise in the age at marriage
- Increasing urbanization and industrialization
- Compulsory education
- Social security measures
- Planned parenthood
- Change in the tax structure

Recreation

210. State the population policies in India.

- Antenatal policy which aims at discouraging the growth of the population
- Distributional policy which deals with the distributional or imbalance of the population

211. Mention the measures to control population explosion.

- Incentives versus disincentives
- Kerala's model substantial investment in health and education
- Region wise approach implementation of family planning program
- Searching for new contraceptives
- Increase in marriage age
- Economic development
- Role of NGO'S

212. Define drug abuse.

It is defined as "self administration of a drug for non-medical reasons" Drug abuse is the use of illicit drug or misuse of legitimate drug resulting into physical or psychological harm

213. Define drug addiction.

It is characteristic by a "compulsion to use the drug, a tendency to increase the dose, psychic, physical dependence and detrimental effects of the individuals and on society"

214. List down the abusal drugs.

- Alcohol
- Sedatives or depressants
- Stimulants

- Hallucinogens
- Narcotics
- Nicotine

215. Mention the causes of drug abuse.

- Psychological causes- Anxiety and frustration
- Social causes-Social inadequacy
- Physiological causes Heightening sexual experiences
- Other causes -Lack of motivation, environmental pressure, peer pressure, dominant sub culture, authoritarianism, emotional disturbance, sexual freedom.

216. List down the measures to control drug abuse.

- Imparting the evil effects of drug abuse
- Changing physician attitudes
- Understanding follow up studies
- Giving deterrent punishment
- Role of parent and teachers
- Multidimensional drug control programme

217. Define juvenile delinquency.

CCB Mamonia writes as, the phrase " juvenile delinquency used to cover any kind of deviant behavior of children which violets normative rules, understanding or expectation group of social system."

218. List down the causes of juvenile delinquency.

- Broken homes
- Poverty
- Companions and gangs
- Beggary
- School dissatisfaction
- Emotional problems
- Mental deficiency in delinquency

219. List the remedies for juvenile delinquency.

Two methods

- Preventive
- Rehabilitative or curative

Government as well as private agencies must work hand in hand with all sincerity and seriousness to find an effective remedy for the problem of juvenile delinquency.

220. How do you prevent juvenile delinquency?

- Creating and inspiring a tem to work
- Giving proper training to control delinquency
- Establishing child guidance clinic
- Educating the family
- Giving proper assistance to under privileged children
- Improving the social environment
- The problems of beggary and poverty are to be removed

221. List the legislative measures to prevent juvenile delinquency.

Legislative measures to prevent juvenile delinquency are:

- Apprentices act of 1850
- Reformatory schools act of 1897
- Provisional in the criminal code
- Children acts
- Juvenile smoking acts
- Suppression of immoral traffic acts
- Probation of offenders act
- Borstal schools acts for adolescents

222. Mention the institutions to rehabilitate juvenile delinquents.

- Juvenile courts
- Remand homes
- Certified schools
- Auxiliary homes
- Foster homes
- Reformatory schools
- Borstal institutions

- Fat persons institutions and uncared children institutions

223. Who is a beggar?

A beggar is one who ask for alms or charity or performs such actions which derive sympathy from others and who give something in return

224. List the types of beggars.

- Able bodied – Adult beggars
- Able bodied – Child beggars
- Heredity beggars
- Sick or diseased beggars
- Physical disabled
- Mentally retarded
- Old and incapable people
- Religious mendicants

225. Mention the causes of beggary.

- Economic causes (poverty, lack of employment/under employment)
- Social causes (lack of parental control, Family disorganization, Breakdown of joint family)
- Biological causes: (sickness, physical or mental defects and old age)
- Religious causes

226. Classify unemployment.

- Seasonal Unemployment
- Agricultural Unemployment
- Technological Unemployment
- Industrial Unemployment
- Cyclical Unemployment
- Educational Unemployment
- Temporary Unemployment
- Voluntary Unemployment

227. List the causes of unemployment.

- Population, division and fragmentation of agricultural land
- Seasonal land of agriculture
- Lack of literacy
- Educational and technical training
- Fatalistic attitudes
- Poverty, frustration
- Chronic ailments

228. Point out the evil effects of unemployment.

- Personal disorganization
- Family disorganization
- Social disorganization
- Irreparable economic losses

229. Mention remedial measures and suggestions to control unemployment.

- Population control
- Promoting economic development
- Promoting agricultural development
- Industrial development
- Education reforms
- Five year plans

230. Mention government schemes to remove the problem of unemployment.

- Integrated Rural Development Programme (IRDP)
- National Rural Employment Programme (NREP)
- Rural Landless Employment Guarantee (RLEP) Programme
- Training Rural Youth For Self Employment (TRYSEM)
- Jawahar Rozar Yojana (JRY)
- Minimum needs programme (MNP)
- Self Employment programme for the urban poor
- Nehru Rozar Yojana (NRY)

231. Mention the consequences of child marriage.

- Irresponsibility
- Adverse effects on health
- Overpopulation
- Female illiteracy
- Low sex ratio
- Child widows

- Hinders personality development
- Inability to select proper mate

232. Define prostitution.

Prostitution is the worst form of exploitation of women. It may be defined as the practice of indulging in promiscuous sexual relations for money

233. List the causes for prostitution.

Economic causes

Social norms-widow remarriage, unhappy marital life, industrialization and urbanization.

234. Mention remedies for prostitution.

- Proper health education about social, moral and STD hygiene
- Suppuration of immoral traffic in women and girls act was enacted, under which it was declared a legal offence to keep brothels, to enter girls and women's and use them for prostitution
- Establishment of rescue homes and shelter for the women in prostitution
- Rehabilitation : find them useful work

235. What are the evil effects of dowry?

- Dowry leads to cruelty towards brides
- Suicide
- ncompatible marriage
- Constants quarrels
- Low status of women

236. List the types of child labour.

- Domestic nonmonetary work
- Non domestic nonmonetary work
- Wage labour
- Bonded labour

237. List the causes of child labour.

- Economic causes
- Cheap labour
- Total failure of governmental machinery and lack of public awareness

238. Specify the consequences of child labour

- The emotional tie between children and their parents are disturbed
- Exploitation of children
- It affects their health

239. Enlist the remedies to the problems of child labour.

- Eradication of poverty
- Providing minimum and fare wages to parents
- Extension of free compulsory education
- Strict enforcement and job security
- Programmatic and multi dimensional
- Committed administration
- Collective responsibility

240. What is youth unrest?

Unrest (student power) seems to have an anti-establishment and a revolutionary tone.

E.g.: A quarrel between the staff of the bus transport and a group of students

241. List the causes of youth unrest.

- Improper socialization and family problems
- Political, social and economic inequalities
- Defective educational system
- Unemployment
- Corrupt
- Misuse of student power by the politicians
- Communication gap
- Influences of movie

242. List the types of youth unrest.

Four forms of youth unrest according to Myron are:

- Political activities and movements
- Students agitation for educational causes
- Agitation against non-university authorities
- Spontaneous student agitation

243. State the remedies for youth unrest.

- System of education
- Employment opportunities
- Provision for leisure time activities
- Economic difficulties –earn while you learn
- Discipline
- Able leadership
- Role of political parties
- Student is participation

244. Define crime.

Crime is an act forbidden by the law of the land and for which penalty is prescribed-C. Darrow Crime is a form of anti-social behavior that has violated public sentiment to such an extent as to be forbidden by statue

245. What is white color crime?

The crime committed by the upper strata of society in their business and professional practices -E.g.: telecom scan, sugar scan, black mark elegy

246. What are the causes of crime?

The causes are biological, social, psychological and economic

- Biological causes: It may include insanity, physical disability, defective glandular and nervous system
- Psychological causes: Neurosis, psychopathy and emotional instability
- Social causes: Conflict, lack of education and cultural lag
- Economic causes: Poverty, unemployment, poor natural resources and inflation

247. How will we solve the problem of crime?

Only a completely removed society, one in which there is no capitalism, can solve the problem of crime

248. Name child welfare programmes.

Child welfare programmes are: Crèches, day care center, early childhood welfare center and pattern integrated family welfare programme, national award for child welfare, celebration of children's day, midday meal scheme, children's film society, balbharoans, children's libraries, children's book trust.

249. Mention social welfare measures for scheduled caste and other backward communities.

- National overseas scholarships for enabling the candidate belonging to scheduled caste and scheduled tribe to go abroad for higher education
- Special representation in the Lok sabha and the state Vidhan sabhas to scheduled castes and tribes
- Women welfare – Marriage scholarship
- Reservation in service and education

250. Name the social welfare organisations for women in India.

- Indian red cross
- Rotary club and lions club
- Indian prostitutes welfare society
- Family planning associations of India
- Indian council for women welfare
- Indian council for social welfare
- National federation of Indian women
- Human rights organization
- Mahila mandals
- Kasturba Gandhi trust
- Kamala Nehru memorial trust

251. What is STEP scheme?

It is known as step to render support to women's employment in various sector such as agriculture, dairying, animal husbandry, fish's khadai and village industries, handicrafts and scripture

252. Explain mahila mandals.

The scheme of welfare extension project

started in 1954 to provide basic minimum services to women and children compressing balwadies, maternity and child health services, literacy and social education for women, arts and crafts centers and recreational facilities in the rural areas was handed over to voluntary organization

253. Mention the functions of family life institute.

The major functions of Counselling services are family life education for the maladjusted spouses, parents, unmarried youths and teenagers of unsettled and depressed mind, child school drop outs

254. What are the problems of old age?

The old age people suffer from numerous familial, social, economic and psychological problems

255. Specify the welfare facilities for old age.

- Reasonable amount of old age pension
- Free medical care and medical insurance
- Housing facilities in the form of old age homes
- Recreational facilities to relieve their loneliness

256. Name two voluntary organizations concerned with care and welfare of the aged

- Help-age India
- Age-care India

257. What is "Adopt a granny scheme?

It is intended to provide rehabilitation at the door steps to the elder living under poverty line. The scheme is sponsored by help age international and under the scheme, the aged are provided with 64 pounds per year.by their sponsors overseas in order to meet their daily needs.

258. How to deal with the aged?

Effective treatment of the older people suffering from mental and other problem requires, comprehensive use of medical psychological and sociological procedures

259. What is Jawahar Rozgar Yojna (JRY)?

It was introduced in the month of April 1989 with the intention of helping at least one month of each of the poorest family by providing employment for about 50 to 100 days in a year at his own work place or residential area

260. List the rights of women.

- Equal educational right
- Equal employment right
- Right to vote
- Right to marry
- Right to divorce

261. List the rights of children.

- Right to be loved
- Right to nutritious food and good health
- Right to education
- Right to get his/her nationality
- Right to relief in case of natural calamities
- Right to get others attention in distress

262. Enlist the objectives of ICDS.

- To improve the nutritional and health status of children in the age group of 0 to 6 years
- To lay the foundations for proper psychological, physical and social development of the child
- To reduce the mortality, morbidity, malnutrition and school dropout
- Supplementary nutrition is given to 0 -6 years
- Immunization of the children below 6 years
- Non-formal preschool education
- Nutrition education and health education